YOUR FOOD-ALLERGIC CHILD

a parent's guide

Janet E. Meizel

Foreword by Frederic Speer, M.D.

Mills & Sanderson, Publishers

Bedford, Massachusetts

1988

LIBRARY OF CONGRESS

Library of Congress Cataloging-in-Publication Data

Meizel, Janet E., 1944-
Your food-allergic child : a parent's guide / Janet E. Meizel.
p. cm.
Bibliography: p.
Includes indes.
ISBN 0-938179-16-0 (pbk.) : $9.95
1. Food allergy in children. 2. Food allergy in children--Diet
therapy--Recipes. 3. Food--Analysis--Tables. I. Title.
RJ386.5.M45 1988
618.92'9750654--dc19   88-23592
                                                        CIP
Printed and Bound in the United States of America

Cover design by Lyrl Ahern.
Printed and Manufactured by Bawden Printing, Inc., Eldridge, IA.

CONTENTS

REFERENCE MATERIALS

Foreword

Medical students complain that clinical courses tend to emphasize diagnosis to the neglect of treatment. The answer they are given, and the lesson they learn later for themselves, is that diagnosis is much the more difficult of the two disciplines and by far the most important; diagnostic failure inevitably leads to treatment failure. But once the diagnosis is established, modern treatment is so standardized that prescribing treatment is relatively easy.

The treatment of food allergy, as far as the physician is concerned is remarkably simple. All he needs to do is hand the patient, or, in the case of children, the parents, a list of foods that must be avoided. But for those who must provide a diet free of these foods, treatment may be most difficult.

Those who are called on to carry out this task are greatly in need of expert guidance. This is supplied in this readable and practical book. The author explores every facet of food-allergen avoidance, discussing food sources, biological food relationships, nutritional guidance, sources of drug allergens, commercial sources of hypo-allergenic foods, and recipes for all sorts of nutritious and appealing meat and vegetable dishes. This book is useful for readers of all degrees of commitment to food avoidance. Those whose commitment does not go beyond making use of the recipes will find their needs met. Those who want to go deeper into the subject will also find their needs met. Mrs. Meizel is to be commended for providing so complete a guide in this important type of allergy.

Frederic Speer, M.D.

Acknowledgments

The author gratefully acknowledges the following sources of information used in this book:

El Molino Mills
Ener-G Foods, Inc.
The California Turkey Industry Board
The California Apricot Advisory Board
Dr. K. H. Steinkraus et al. of Cornell University, for permitting me to use the method of making soy milk which they developed.
Watt and Merill, *Composition of Foods*, United States Department of Agriculture, 1985.
Furia, Thomas E., *CRC Handbook of Food Additives*, Chemical Rubber Company, Ohio, 1972.
Crow, W. B., *A Synopsis of Biology*, 2nd Edition, Wright and Sons, Bristol, 1964.
Frederic Speer for his list of food families.
All the companies who supplied me with their catalogs and product content lists.

Special thanks are due Frederic Speer, M.D. and Helen Klevickis, M.D. for their help and encouragement.

Introduction

Advances in the fields of immunology, allergy, and other areas of medicine, have shown that many disorders are due to adverse reactions to specific foods or food additives. These normally harmless substances produce ill effects by a variety of means, some of which are not completely understood.

Primary among these reactions is the classic allergic response, during which the following happens:

1. The body produces elevated levels of an "allergic" antibody (IgE) in the blood. This antibody is directed against specific food proteins to which the patient is exposed.

2. On subsequent ingestion of this food, the antibody combines with the food protein.

3. A series of reactions leads to the release of substances which provoke the allergic response. It is the body's reaction to these chemicals which results in the symptoms we recognize as an allergy. These symptoms may vary, but frequently include:

coughing	wheezing
generalized swelling	hives
stuffy nose	headaches
vomiting	fatigue
nasal discharge	irritability
diarrhea	bedwetting
colic	shock
hearing loss due to middle middle ear infections	rashes

There are several ways in which a food allergy is discovered:

Observation. This consists of simply noticing the onset of symptoms after a food is eaten.

Allergy tests. Unfortunately, not all responses to foods are IgE-mediated. Because of this, the standard scratch tests (skin tests) based on this mechanism are not always reliable and some tests may show negative results even though the patient is exhibiting symptoms.

Elimination diet. At present the most effective method of discovering a food allergy, the elimination diet is prescribed and supervised by a physician trained in allergy.

During an elimination diet, the patient is actively involved in both the diagnostic and treatment phases of his problem. Once the symptom-causing foods are discovered, it is usually left to the patient to avoid them, causing a sense of panic in even the most calm parents. (My child is allergic to milk, eggs, grains, and beef. What CAN he eat?)

You will now become a "rare-foods" expert and a gourmet cook. It is amazing how many different meals you can concoct from a few basic ingredients. Varied combinations of foods, cooking methods, and textures can make even a severely limited diet quite palatable. And if you are adventurous, you can try foods from many other countries or regions that require ingredients different from those which cause your child's problems.

The recipe section of this book has been indexed to show which recipes can be used in different diets and combinations, and food tables are provided so you can devise a well-balanced diet. Relationships among the foods and products are indicated to help you avoid the cross reactions which often occur among foods of the same family.

IN THE KITCHEN

After purchasing the foods which your child can tolerate (see the "Resources" section for information on where to buy some of the more difficult-to-find items), the next step is preparation. If there are several people in your family and one or more of them must have a special diet, here are some ways of making food preparation easier:

Cook food in large batches, then seal and freeze individual portions in cooking bags or glass jars. If you use glass jars and intend to reheat the food in a microwave oven, be sure that the jars are capable of withstanding the change in temperature. Otherwise, use wide-mouth jars and remove the food by placing the jar under warm water for a minute. Then cook the food in another container. Freezing is an ideal method for preserving food as it does not permit spoilage or growth of mold. Some foods can be kept frozen longer than others, so be sure to put dates on all your labels.

Other things to think about when organizing your kitchen to cook for someone who is food allergic:

1. There exists such a wide variety of cooking utensils and equipment of varied compositions that suitable ones are easy to find. There are some points to consider when you are purchasing them, however. Glass and stainless steel cookware are the easiest

to clean, having the least porous surfaces. Cast iron cookware may leach a tiny amount of iron into an iron-poor diet, but its rough surface must be very carefully scrubbed clean of offending foods before being used to cook for the food-allergic member of the family.

2. An exhaust fan over the stove is essential since some foods have fumes which may act as triggers for allergic reactions (eggs and fish are frequently the culprits). You will need to clean the filters often. Thorough cleaning is also important for refrigerators and cupboards to avoid dust or the growth of mold in the food. I have found that the new technique of coating some vegetables for longer shelf-life at the supermarket makes it necessary to use the food sooner.

3. Foods for different diets should be kept separated. When our children were small, we kept their cookies and crackers in a separate "cookie drawer" within their reach, so that they would not confuse them with anyone else's. A bonus of this method was that the children grew proud of their ability to reach their own snacks, when given permission. This seemed to soften the imposition of the diet and reinforce the idea of which foods they could and could not have.

One last thing

If a child has a life-threatening allergy to a food, be sure to make it totally unavailable to him. If some time has passed since he/she has had a severe allergic episode, a child may forget and be tempted to try the offending food. If you must have the food in the house, be sure to label it with a warning in case a baby-sitter or other temporary caretaker forgets the restrictions. Even though our children are now capable of remembering their own diets, we still keep foods for different diets separated. In a hurry, anyone can make a mistake.

I hope you enjoy the recipes. With practice and a little planning, allergy cooking is easily managed and will become just another part of life rather than a major concern.

Helpful Terms

Jewish dietary law separates food into three categories, and many products at the grocery store are marked this way.

Dairy contains milk or milk products, but cannot contain any other animal product.

Meat contains animal product, but the only ones permitted are beef, lamb, fish, or poultry (no pork).

Pareve contains neither meat nor dairy products of any sort. (For example, Mocha Mix, Tofutti and sorbets are pareve. They substitute for cream and ice cream.) *Pareve u* indicates that the product is certified Kosher by the Union of Orthodox Jewish Congregations of America.

CHILDREN'S SPECIAL

INFANTS

Scientists have discovered at least one specific gene involved in the transmission of allergic tendencies from one generation to the next. If you or your spouse has allergies, your children have a greater chance of developing allergic problems than if neither of you are affected. There are some things you can do to at least delay the onset of symptoms and give the baby's digestive system more time to develop. (Some physicians feel that the younger infant's less-developed digestive system allows more antibody-producing material to enter the baby's bloodstream, beginning the allergic process.)

Most authorities recommend that the mother nurse the baby if at all possible. No known cases of allergy to mother's milk have been found. It is wise, however, to keep track of what the mother eats. Some of the protein which the mother ingests can pass through her milk and cause symptoms in the baby. For example, if the mother eats fish and after nursing notices that the baby has more colic than usual, or has diarrhea, or is unusually stuffy, it is a good idea for her not to eat that same type of fish during the months she is nursing. This applies to all foods — and even to vitamins and medication which the mother might take. For questions about medication, consult the physician who prescribed it, or an allergist. (See Reference section for lists of ingredients in medications.)

Physicians who deal extensively with allergic babies often recommend that they not be given solid food too early, and that once solid food is given, the introduction should be gradual. Introducing each food separately, with ample time between additions, makes it much easier to detect any existing sensitivities. It is much easier to do this with an infant than to try to put a school-age child on an elimination diet when he already has strong opinions about foods that he does or doesn't like.

It is also important to keep the baby's diet simple. By this I mean that each food given to the infant should have as few ingredients as possible. Some of the prepared baby foods contain many ingredients, which make careful label-reading a "must" for the parents of either an allergic baby or one who is suspected of having allergies.

1

Perhaps the most important hint for parents is to choose a physician with whom you have good communication, with whom you are comfortable, and most important, who is knowledgeable in the field of allergy. It is a relatively new field, and many physicians have not received sufficient training in diagnosing the less frequent manifestations of allergic disease. If you feel that you are not receiving adequate assistance with your baby, seek more qualified help.

TODDLERS

Toddlers learn everything very quickly, and it is amazing to see the level of responsibility a two-or-three-year-old can accept for her own diet. If a child has had several allergic episodes, she will usually be willing to avoid the things she associates with that discomfort, and some gentle reinforcement by parents will do wonders. For example, when the offending food is offered, simply saying "that makes your tummy hurt" or "that makes you wheeze" or "that makes you itch" gives the child a direct association which can easily be remembered between the food and a symptom.

At this stage, if the toddler is cared for at home, her opportunities to make dietary mistakes are limited, and most playmates' mothers are willing to make the necessary provisions for snacks. If this is not possible, however, it makes good sense for the toddler to bring her own refreshments.

PRESCHOOL AGE

When your child is a bit older and actually plays with other children or goes to nursery school, sharing becomes a major theme in his life. Protecting him from the foods to which he is allergic becomes more complicated. Sometimes it is a good idea to prepare a snack for the entire group so that the allergic child does not constantly feel stigmatized. There will still be some rough moments. A lunchbox is a real status symbol for this group, and often several children will bring them to nursery school or to play group. Your child may be the first to actually use the lunchbox for carrying food and a beverage, and may view carrying it as a privilege.

It is important that the teacher or day-care mother be aware of any dietary limitations. A major part of the nursery school curriculum includes experimenting with the five senses, including both taste and smell. If a child is violently allergic to wheat, the teacher must understand that it is not appropriate to allow him to taste salt by licking it from a pretzel, simply because the others are eating pretzels. It may help to discuss alternatives with the teacher before a planned activity.

Often "sense" themes are carried over into snack time in nursery school, and often create problems. It may be quite difficult for a small child allergic to orange juice to associate it with the "green juice" teacher made by adding blue food coloring to the juice of an orange. Both the teacher and parents need to be aware that there is little abstract reasoning at this age. The child will not or can not always stop to evaluate a new situation, and instead relies heavily on the judgment of a trusted adult.

There are other situations at nursery school which may provoke food-allergy problems. Here is one of the most popular playdough recipes for school use:

Generic Playdough

1 cup (wheat) flour   1 cup water
1/2 cup salt   Food coloring
2 tablespoons oil

Mix dry ingredients. Mix water and coloring. Then add oil and water to dry ingredients and stir over medium heat until stiff.

Playing with this medium, assisting in its manufacture, or even being in the room where it is being mixed can cause problems for a wheat-allergic child. This problem may be avoided by asking the teacher to use commercially prepared playdough or by providing the school with it. If the school budget does not allow for this purchase and you don't want to supply it for your child's class, this formula for a hardening playdough is on the Argo cornstarch package.

Cornstarch Playdough

1 cup Argo cornstarch   2 cups baking soda

Mix the cornstarch and baking soda in a saucepan. Add 1 1/2 cups cold water and heat, stirring, until it reaches a "mashed-potato" consistency. Turn out on a plate. Cover with a damp cloth and cool. It can then be kneaded like dough. *Author's note:* Color may be added while stirring.

Commercial glue or paste can substitute easily for flour and water paste. If the children are making papier-mache constructions, rice flour and water make a good binding liquid in which to soak the paper strips.

Birthdays are important celebrations in nursery school, and many children bring a treat for the class. Usually the teacher will ask parents for the dates of birthdays, and armed with a copy of this list, you can send a treat with the child on the appropriate day. If the school has a freezer, it is a good idea to keep a reserve supply of home-made cupcakes, cookies, or even ice pops there, since parents have been known to surprise teachers by bringing unexpected snacks.

ELEMENTARY AGE

Most of the preceeding suggestions are appropriate for elementary school. However there are a few additional complications in this setting due to the fact that elementary schools are somewhat more impersonal than nursery schools.

The first problem encountered by parents of allergic children is how to notify the teacher of the child's problem without making an issue of it. Some school districts will not permit the parents to know the teacher's name before the first day of school. Other districts do not give the teachers complete student records to avoid "prejudicing" the teacher. In both cases, you should try to convince school officials of the necessity of changing these regulations. A complete list of restrictions and emergency procedures should be given to the teacher before he/she comes in contact with the child, for the most effective teaching situation. Then the teacher should be allowed to ask you any questions which he/she feels are pertinent. Most teachers are anxious to help their students learn to cope, and this includes helping children develop a positive attitude about whatever problems they may have.

Once in a while, you will find a teacher who "does not believe" in allergy (there are even physicians who share this attitude). At the other extreme is the teacher who creates a stressful situation by placing too much emphasis on a child's "handicap." Both extremes cause additional problems, and it is imperative to speak to the teacher and correct the situation. If the problem cannot be solved by this method, change the child's class placement.

4

Due to budget cuts, many schools are without nurses, and other personnel are not allowed to administer medication in any form. While an unusually responsible child may be given her own medication and instructions for taking it, many schools object. It is often better to provide the school with a list of several alternate adults who may be called in to take responsibility for administering medication to the child. If the allergy is so severe that there is a time element involved for successful treatment, be sure that all school personnel are informed. A copy of emergency procedures, in the order in which they must be carried out, should be attached to the student's permanent record and to the emergency card which is always kept in the school office.

Many elementary schools hold parties for the holidays (usually Halloween, winter vacation, Valentine's Day, and year-end) and an important feature of the parties is food. The teacher will provide you with the dates and times so that your child can have a treat along with the others. Cookies cut in special designs and rock candy (crystallized sugar) are usually acceptable treats. Some teachers even prefer fruit (any tolerated fruit, cut up, will do) and fancy vegetables. Most children like to share their things with the class, and I have found that bringing apple juice (or another juice) or fruit makes the children feel very good about themselves and their ability to contribute.

TRAVELING

Another area which frequently presents problems to parents of food-allergic children is what to do when travelling. While most restaurants will make accommodations for babies and toddlers, they are not always receptive to a school-age child bringing his own food. However, a simple request before entering the restaurant with the child usually suffices, and I have found most people to be willing to assist. When possible, I ask if they can prepare a plate for the child with what she can eat, explaining the reason. Naturally, we usually go to restaurants where they can provide us with this courtesy. We also travel with a supply of those foods the children can tolerate tucked into an ice chest "just in case." When traveling by air with an infant, I have found it advisable to be prepared with enough ready-to-serve formula for the length of the trip plus at least two feedings. If you must make up the formula at home, place it in a cold pack and carry it aboard with you. You wouldn't want to lose it in the luggage bay of a 747. This method also avoids the possibility of any problems arising from use of the local water.

Ordering a special meal on an airliner is quite risky, so it is much safer to provide your own. After requesting a special meal on one cross-country flight, my three-year-old was served her chicken and vegetables at 8:00 A.M. and nothing else was available for the rest of the day. Luckily we had brought other food with us, just in case our test run didn't work.

Most hotels and motels have rooms equipped with small refrigerators, or, if they don't, are willing to let you replace the ice in a cooler. Many also have hot-plates on which you can at least prepare breakfast in the room. Vacation is not the time to experiment with foods. Most restauranteurs are glad to answer questions about food preparation. For example: if your child loves french-fried potatoes, in what fat are they fried? (The answer may be peanut, corn, soy, sunflower or safflower oil, lard, etc.) If your child is sensitive to sulfites, is the salad, potato or fruit dipped in a sulfite solution to keep it fresh-looking? It might be safer to settle for broiled chicken and a baked potato.

Take with you any medication your child normally takes and enough of any emergency medication which the doctor recommends. *Don't rely on a written prescription.* Finding an open pharmacy in a strange place or getting an out-of-town prescription filled can be difficult. We also have the children wear a Medic-Alert™ tag on a necklace or bracelet when we travel. In case of an accident, each tag lists their major sensitivities and has a phone number (with instructions to call collect) from which in an emergency any physician can get all the child's pertinent information. While we have never needed to use the tags, I am much more comfortable knowing that the children wear them.

Since food-related activities are so numerous in the pre-school and elementary school years, it is very important to find ways to keep a child from feeling different. One of the best ways is to provide him with enough food substitutes so that he doesn't feel left out, and include the child in as many of the family meals as possible.

In this chapter, you will find many children's favorites recipes and alternative ingredients to substitute for allergenic ones. Included in these recipes are some commercially available products, so that, when possible, these foods can be made at home. If

6

these products are not available locally, the manufacturers' addresses are listed in the Resources section so that you can write to them or to the distributer for purchasing information.

To begin at the beginning, I have listed the various milk-free formulas currently available, their contents and restrictions. This is not meant to take the place of medical consultation, but to make the search for a formula easier. Since diagnosis of food allergy relies to a great extent on parental observation, comparison of a baby's reaction to a different formula (colic, irritability, stuffiness, digestive problems, etc.) will help to single out the offending elements.

NOTES ON FORMULAS

In 1980, the Federal Government passed the Infant Formula Act, which regulates the minimum amounts of nutrients which must be present in all infant formulas. (Public Law 96-359) These are the requirements as stated in that Act.:

Nutrient	Recommended Minimum (per 100 kcal)	
Vitamin A	250.0	I.U.
Vitamin D	40.0	I.U.
Vitamin E	0.7	I.U.
Vitamin K	4.0	mcg
Vitamin C	8.0	mcg
Thiamine	40.0	mcg
Riboflavin	60.0	mcg
Vitamin B_1	35.0	mcg
Folic Acid	4.0	mcg
Vitamin B_2	.15	mcg
Pantothenic Acid	300.0	mcg
Biotin	1.5	mcg
Calcium	50.0	mg
Phosphorus	25.0	mg
Magnesium	6.0	mg
Iron	0.15	mg
Iodine	5.09	mcg
Zinc	0.5	mcg
Copper	60.0	mcg
Manganese	5.0	mcg
Sodium	20.0	mg

Nutrient	Recommended Minimum
Potassium	80.0 mg
Chloride	55.0 mg

Remember that these are requirements for INFANT formulas. If your child must continue on one of these formulas, consult a nutritionist who can determine whether your child's diet is adequate for growth and maintenance of health needs. At different stages of development, a child's needs change. If a nutritionist is not available, most large city hospitals have dieticians on staff who are used to formulating special diets, and can help you to choose a nutritionally appropriate one for your child.

It is also possible that due to other problems one or more of these formulas is not suitable for your infant. A conference with both pediatrician and allergist can solve some of these problems.

RCF Ross Carbohydrate-Free Soy Protein Formula Base (Ross Laboratories, Columbus, Ohio 43216)

Ingredients: (Pareve u) water, soy protein isolate, coconut oil, soy oil, calcium phosphates (mono-and tribasic), potassium citrate, potassium chloride, carageenan, mono-and diglycerides, soy lecithin, magnesium chloride, calcium carbonate, L-methionine, ascorbic acid, sodium chloride, choline chloride, zinc sulfate, vitamin concentrate (alpha-tocopheryl acetate, Vitamin A palmitate, phylloquinone, and Vitamin D), niacinamide, calcium pantothenate, cupric sulfate, thiamine chloride hydrochloride, riboflavin, pyridoxine hydrochloride, folic acid, biotin, and cyanocobalamin.

Approximate Analysis	Standard Dilution (wt/liter)*
Protein	20.0 g
Fat	36.0 g
Carbohydrate	**
Calories per 100 ml.	**
Minerals (ash)	3.8 g
Calcium	0.70 g
Phosphorus	0.50 g
Sodium	0.30 g
Potassium	0.71 g
Chloride	0.53 g
Magnesium	0.05 g

Approximate Analysis	Standard Dilution	
Iron	1.5	mg

(This product is deficient in iron; an additional 5.3 mg. of iron per liter should be supplied from other sources.)

Zinc	5.0	mg
Copper	0.50	mg
Iodine	0.10	mg
Manganese	0.20	mg
Vitamin A	2500	I.U.
Vitamin D	400	I.U.
Vitamin E	17	I.U.
Vitamin C	55	mg
Thiamin	0.40	mg
Riboflavin	0.60	mg
Vitamin B	0.40	mg
Niacin	9.0	(mg equiv.)
Folic Acid	0.10	mg
Vitamin B_{12}	3.0	mcg
Pantothenic Acid	5.0	mg
Biotin	30	mcg
Vitamin K	0.15	mg

*Standard dilution is one part RCF formula base to one part prescribed carbohydrate and water solution.

**Varies depending on quantity of carbohydrate and water used. If carbohydrate is not added to this product, a 1:1 dilution with water provides approximately 12 kcal per fluid ounce (40 kcal/100 ml).

ISOMIL formula (Ross Laboratories, Columbus, Ohio 43216)

Ingredients: (Pareve) water, corn syrup, sucrose, soy protein isolate, soy oil, coconut oil, modified corn starch, minerals (calcium phosphate tribasic, potassium citrate, potassium chloride, magnesium chloride, sodium chloride, ferrous sulfate, zinc sulfate, cupric sulfate, manganese sulfate, potassium iodide), mono- and diglycerides, soy lecithin, vitamins (ascorbic acid, choline chloride, alpha tocopheryl acetate, niacinamide, calcium pantothenate, Vitamin A palmitate, thiamine chloride hydrochloride, riboflavin, pyridoxine hydrochloride, phylloquinone, folic acid, biotin, Vitamin D, cyanocobalamin), L-methionine, and carageenan.

Approximate Analysis	Standard Dilution (wt/liter)*	
Protein	20.0	g
Fat	36.0	g
Carbohydrate	68.0	g
Minerals (ash)	3.8	g
Calcium	0.70	g
Phosphorus	0.50	g
Sodium	0.30	g
Potassium	0.71	g
Chloride	0.53	g
Magnesium	50	mg
Iron	12	mg
Zinc	5.0	mg
Copper	0.50	mg
Iodine	0.10	mg
Manganese	0.20	mg
Vitamin A	2500	I.U.
Vitamin D	400	I.U.
Vitamin E	20	I.U.
Vitamin C	55	mg
Thiamine	0.40	mg
Riboflavin	0.60	mg
Vitamin B_1	0.40	mg
Niacin	9.0	mg equiv.
Folic Acid	0.10	mg
Vitamin B_{12}	3.0	mcg
Pantothenic Acid	5.0	mg
Biotin	30	mcg
Vitamin K_1	0.15	mg
Inisotol	60	mg
Choline	80	mg
Water	901.6	g

Calories per 100 ml.: 68

*Standard dilution is one part concentrated liquid to one part water.

PROSOBEE Milk-Free Formula with Soy Protein Isolate (Mead Johnson and Company Evansville, IN 47721)
Ingredients: Water, corn syrup solids, soy oil, soy protein isolate, coconut oil, tribasic calcium phosphate, lecithin, tribasic potassium citrate, salt, magnesium chloride, L-methionine, calcium

carbonate, carrageenan, Vitamin A palmitate, ergocalciferol, di-alpha-tocopheryl acetate, sodium ascorbate, folic acid, thiamine hydrochloride, riboflavin, niacinamide, pyridoxine hydrochloride, cyanocobalamin, biotin, calcium pantothenate, phytonadione, choline chloride, inisotol, potassium iodide, ferrous sulfate, cupric sulfate, zinc sulfate, manganese sulfate.

Approximate Analysis	Standard Dilution*
Protein	2 g per 100 ml
Fat	3.6 g per 100 ml
Carbohydrate	6.9 g per 100 ml
Minerals (ash)	0.4 g per 100 ml
Kilocalories	20 per fl. oz.

Vitamins and Minerals (per quart)

Vitamin A	2000	I.U.
Vitamin D	400	I.U.
Vitamin E	10	I.U.
Vitamin C (ascorbic acid)	52	mg
Folic Acid (folacin)	100	mcg
Thiamine	0.5	mg
Niacin	8	mg
Vitamin B_6	0.4	mg
Vitamin B_{12}	2	mcg
Biotin	2	mcg
Pantothenic Acid	3	mg
Vitamin K_1	100	mcg
Choline	50	mcg
Inisotol	30	mg
Calcium	600	mg
Phosphorus	475	mg
Iodine	65	mcg
Iron	12	mg
Magnesium	70	mg
Copper	0.6	mg
Zinc	5	mg
Manganese	0.2	mg
Chloride	520	mg
Potassium	780	mg
Sodium	275	mg

*Standard dilution = equal amounts of Prosobee concentrate and water.

Mead Johnson states that Prosobee is lactose/sucrose-free.

ISOMIL SF Sucrose-Free Soy Protein Formula (Ross Laboratories, Columbus, OH 43216)

Ingredients: (Pareve) Water, corn syrup solids, soy protein isolate, soy oil, coconut oil, minerals (calcium phosphate tribasic, potassium citrate, potassium chloride, magnesium chloride, calcium carbonate, sodium chloride, ferrous sulfate, zinc sulfate, cupric sulfate, potassium iodide), mono-and diglycerides, soy lecithin, vitamins (ascorbic acid, choline chloride, alpha-tocopheryl acetate, niacinamide, calcium pantothenate, Vitamin A palmitate, thiamine chloride hydrochloride, riboflavin, pyridoxine hydrochloride, phylloquinone, folic acid, biotin, Vitamin D_3, cyanocobalamin, and L-methionine. For approximate analysis see ISOMIL.

NURSOY Soy Protein Formula (Wyeth Laboratories, Inc., Philadelphia, PA 19101)

Ingredients: Water, sucrose, oleo, coconut, oleic (safflower) and soybean oils, soy protein isolate, monobasic sodium phosphate, potassium citrate, calcium carbonate, magnesium chloride, calcium hydroxide, soy lecithin, calcium chloride, L-methionine, dibasic calcium phosphate, sodium chloride, calcium carrageenan, potassium bicarbonate, ferrous zinc, manganese and cupric sulfates, potassium iodide, ascorbic acid, choline chloride, alpha tocopheryl acetate, niacinamide, calcium pantothenate, riboflavin, Vitamin A palmitate, thiamine hydrochloride, pyridoxine hydrochloride, beta-carotene, phytonadione, folic acid, biotin, activated 7-dehydrocholesterol, cyanocobalamin.

Approximate Analysis	Standard Dilution(W/V)*
Protein	2.1%
Fat	3.6%
Carbohydrate	6.9%
Ash	0.35%
Water	87.0%
Crude Fiber	not more than 0.01%
Calories	20 per fl. oz.

Vitamins and Minerals (per quart)

Vitamin A	2500	I.U.
Vitamin D_3	400	I.U.
Vitamin E	9	I.U.
Vitamin K_1	0.1	mg
Vitamin C (ascorbic acid)	55	mg
Thiamine	0.67	mg
Riboflavin	1	mg
Vitamin B_6	0.4	mg
Vitamin B_{12}	2	mcg
Niacin	9.5	(mg equiv.)
Pantothenic Acid	3	mg
Folic Acid	50	mcg
Choline	85	mg
Biotin	35	mcg
Calcium	600	mg
Phosphorus	420	mg
Sodium	190	mg
Potassium	700	mg
Chloride	350	mg
Magnesium	65	mg
Manganese	1	mg
Iron	12	mg
Copper	0.45	mg
Zinc	3.5	mg
Iodine	65	mcg

*Standard dilution is one part concentrated liquid to one part water.

SOYALAC Concentrate Milk-Free Soy Formula for Infants (Loma Linda Foods, Riverside, CA 92515)

Ingredients: (Pareve u) Water, soybean solids, corn syrup, sugar, soy oil, calcium carbonate, soy lecithin, sodium citrate tribasic, calcium phosphate dibasic, calcium citrate tribasic, potassium phosphate dibasic, salt, ascorbic acid, potassium chloride, L-methionine, ferrous sulfate, zinc sulfate, potassium citrate, di-Alpha-Tocopheryl acetate, niacinamide, D-calcium pantothenate, calcium chloride, Vitamin A palmitate, thiamine hydrochloride, riboflavin, cupric sulfate, pyridoxine, hydrochloride, potassium iodide, phytonadione, ergocalciferol, biotin, folic acid, cyanocobalamin.

Approximate Analysis	**Standard Dilution (W/V)**
Protein	2.1%
Fat	3.7%
Minerals (ash)	0.4%
Water	90%
Fiber	0.0%
Calories per fluid ounce	20

Vitamins and Minerals (per quart)

Vitamin A	2000	I.U.
Vitamin D	400	I.U.
Vitamin E	15	I.U.
Vitamin K	50	mcg
Vitamin C	60	mg
Folacin	100	mcg
Thiamine	500	mg
Niacin equivalents	8	mg
Vitamin B_6	400	mg
Vitamin B_{12}	2	mcg
Biotin	50	mcg
Pantothenic Acid	3	mg
Choline	100	mg
Inositol	100	mg
Sodium	330	mg
Potassium	700	mg
Magnesium	70	mg
Calcium	600	mg
Manganese	1	mg
Iron	12	mg
Copper	500	mcg
Zinc	5	mg
Phosphorus	400	mg
Chloride	370	mg
Iodine	45	mcg

*Standard dilution is one part Soyalac concentrate to one part water.

I-SOYALAC Concentrate Corn-Free, Milk-Free, Nutritionally-Balanced Soy Isolate Formula (Loma Linda Foods Riverside, CA 92515)

Ingredients: (Pareve u) Water, sugar, soy oil, soy protein isolate, tapioca dextrin, calcium phosphate dibasic, potassium citrate, soy lecithin, calcium carbonate, potassium chloride, L-methionine, magnesium phosphate dibasic, calcium citrate tribasic, magnesium chloride, ascorbic acid, salt, choline chloride, ferrous sulfate, inositol, zinc sulfate, di-Alpha-Tocopheryl acetate, niacinamide, D-calcium pantothenate, Vitamin A palmitate, cupric sulfate, manganese sulfate, thiamine hydrochloride, riboflavin, pyridoxine hydrochloride, potassium iodide, folic acid, phytonadione, biotin, ergocalciferol, cyanocobalamin.

Vitamins and Minerals (per quart)

Vitamin A	2000	I.U.
Vitamin D	400	I.U.
Vitamin E	15	I.U.
Vitamin K	50	mcg
Vitamin C	60	mg
Folacin	100	mcg
Thiamine	500	mcg
Riboflavin	600	mcg
Niacin equivalents	8	mg
Vitamin B_6	400	mcg
Vitamin B_{12}	2	mcg
Biotin	50	mcg
Pantothenic acid	3	mg
Choline	100	mg
Inositol	100	mg
Sodium	320	mg
Potassium	750	mg
Magnesium	60	mg
Calcium	600	mg
Manganese	500	mcg
Iron	12	mg
Copper	500	mcg
Zinc	5	mg
Phosphorus	400	mg
Chloride	500	mg
Iodine	45	mcg

*Standard dilution is one part I-Soyalac to one part water.

BABY FOOD

When the baby is old enough to try "solid" food, it is advisable to introduce one food at a time. Although commercially prepared baby food is well-labelled, it is very easy to make your own, if necessary. At this stage in a baby's life, "the simpler, the better."

These recipes can be pureed in a blender or forced through a fine sieve until they are smooth. Begin with thoroughly cooked foods as they have been found to be better tolerated than raw ones.

MEAT

1/2 cup cubed cooked meat
4 to 6 tablespoons formula, water, or simple beef broth
(See Beef Stock recipe on Page 102.)

VEGETABLES

1/2 cup cut-up vegetables
4 to 5 tablespoons formula, water, or broth

FRUIT

3/4 cup cooked fruit
2 to 3 tablespoons syrup or juice from fruit

As the baby gets older, you can puree the food to a somewhat coarser consistency (for "junior" food). Many children do not like this texture — especially for meats — but since they are usually learning to pick up small objects, they will enjoy the results of the following recipe. The bright colors make easy targets for small fingers, and the ingredients can be chewed or gummed easily.

JUNIOR ONE-DISH MEAL

1/2 cup cooked rice
1/4 cup pre-cooked soybeans or diced meat
1/4 cup diced carrot
1/4 cup peas

Cook the peas and carrots in a small amount of water. Add the cooked soybeans (or meat) and rice, and serve. If you use instant rice, allow it to absorb the cooking liquid from the vegetables so the vitamins aren't lost.

Small children almost universally love frankfurters. Due to the recent surge of interest in "health foods," you can easily purchase all-beef, no cereal frankfurters in most areas of the United States. Kosher frankfurters are all beef, and the "health food" variety do not contain nitrites. (They are found in the "frozen foods" section of the market.) Recently chicken and turkey frankfurters have also become available, but be sure to read the label, as they sometimes contain the same spices and fats — or cereals — as the usual varieties in order to mimic the taste of the original product. This also occurs in soy frankfurters or sausage. Chicken and turkey frankfurters frequently contain lemon juice to prevent the meat from changing color if they do not contain preservatives.

If you are willing (or find it necessary) to make your own frankfurters, you can purchase casing from a meat supplier, or a butchers' supply house. The most frequently used casings are made of lamb or soy, and by making your own frankfurters you can use the spices which are permitted in your child's diet. Many electric mixers have an "optional" sausage stuffer accessory, which makes sausage-making much easier. If you can't use any available casing, you can roll the meat in cheesecloth and tie it at both ends before cooking to help keep a frankfurter-like shape.

A second juvenile favorite is spaghetti. There are some good substitutes for this too, although the taste isn't exactly the same. In any Oriental food store you can find rice sticks, made of rice flour and water. They are more delicate than their wheat-flour counterpart, and cannot be boiled. To prepare rice sticks, pour boiling water over them and allow them to soak until they are soft. (These are sometimes called Saifun.)

Another noodle is made from mung bean paste, and called Maifun. It is prepared the same way, or soaked and then fried until crisp for traditional Chinese dishes.

A third spaghetti-like product is made from buckwheat flour. It can be found in Korean and Japanese food stores, and prepared differently by bringing water to a boil and then adding the noodles. When the noodles rise to the surface of the water, drain and serve.

Along with rice "spaghetti," you will also find rice noodles of different widths and "rice paper" which is frequently used in Chinese cooking.

Recipes for home-made "fun" (noodles):

RICE SPAGHETTI OR NOODLES I

2 cups rice flour
1/2 teaspoon salt
1/2 teaspoon powdered alum (to prevent sticking)
Oil
2 3/4 cups water

Place the flour on a board and sprinkle with the salt and alum. Blend. Add 3 teaspoons of oil and a little water, gradually, to form a ball of dough. Knead for 10 minutes, until elastic. Place dough in a bowl and add the rest of the water. Mix well and let rest for 1/2 an hour. Place 2 inches of water in a large pot with a steaming rack. Oil a pie pan and pour a thin layer of batter on it. Cover, bring water to a boil and steam on medium heat until set (about 15 minutes). Let cool and roll onto a plate. Cut into desired shape.

BUCKWHEAT NOODLES

4 cups buckwheat flour
2/3 cup cornstarch
1/2 teaspoon salt
Lukewarm water

Sift together the dry ingredients and mix in a little water. Knead thoroughly and roll out thinly on a floured board. Slice to desired width.

For more recipes, see the Recipe section . Other alternatives to wheat-based pasta come from Carlo Erba of Italy and EnerG Foods of Seattle, Washington. The first is distributed under the Aproten brand of Chicago Dietetic Supply, Inc. It comes in four forms: rigatini (like elbow macaroni); Tagliatelle (thin noodles); anellini (ring macaroni for soups, etc.) and semolina (hot cereal). The Aproten noodles are made from cornstarch, tapioca starch, micro-crystalline cellulose and artificial color. They are low protein, contain no gluten and are low in phenylalanine. (See Reference section for address.) Ener-G distributes Aglutella brand noodles, spaghetti and macaroni which contain corn starch, rice starch, potato starch, monoglycerides and carotene. They contain no artificial flavors, colors or binders.

Other vermicelli formulas to be found in Oriental food stores are arrowroot vermicelli and bean thread (made from green beans and potato starch or from green bean starch and water—lungkow vermicelli). These also are soaked in boiling water until pliable.

PLAYGROUP SNACKS

It is easier to substitute apple juice, pear nectar, or apricot nectar (or any other fruit juice) to children accustomed to drinking cow's milk, than to serve soy milk. Soy milk has a distinctive taste and is not likely to be appreciated. The result could be comments which would hurt the feelings of the allergic child.

I have found the best-accepted wheat-egg-milk free snack to be plain rice cakes or rice cakes with jam or almost any other spread. Rice cakes are made from "puffed" rice formed to make a round. (I also break them up to make "popped rice" when popcorn is being served and recently discovered that my daughter's friends with braces appreciate this as they cannot eat popcorn.) Small, salty rice crackers of several types are also available and well accepted by children. Frequently vanilla rice cookies or mixed-flour cookies are well received, as are carob sandwich cookies. (See Recipe section.) Carrots, raisins, celery, or raw, dried or stewed fruit are also popular. Fancy snacks are completely unnecessary at this age, and the most popular treats are those which can be picked up in fingers without much fuss.

SCHOOL LUNCHES

Sometimes a child will choose one favorite lunch which he wants every day (peanut butter and jelly ranks very high with this group), but it is important to vary the foods an allergic child takes in as it is possible to "wear out" a food and begin to develop symptoms from it.

Some suggestions: Put stewed fruit or a portion of stew or casserole in a small thermos dish. Give your child hot soup instead of milk on a cold day, fruit juice, or flavored soy milk for a change (soy milk and honey or carob soy milk).

If you are making a sandwich with rice bread, toast the bread first. Otherwise it has a tendency to fall apart before lunch. Even after toasting, it is still fragile, and wrapping the sandwich in aluminum foil, or using a lunchbox rather than a bag will give it more protection. If you buy small cans of fruit juice, you can freeze them and let them thaw in the lunchbox. This keeps the lunch cool on a hot day while providing a cold drink. If your child cannot eat food from a metal container, glass-lined Thermos bottles are available.

Dried, as well as fresh fruits, provide a good ending to a school lunch. Most health food stores sell dried apricots, prunes, apples, bananas and papayas (some with sulfur and some without). They also sell banana chips and additive-free potato chips. Fruit leather, (dried, pureed fruit) is also a favorite with schoolchildren.

It is especially important to provide your child on a limited diet with something he likes if you hope to avoid the results of "lunch trading," a popular pastime at all schools.

PARTY SPECIALS

Parties are supposed to be fun. They should include all the activities and refreshments, and can be quite a challenge if your child is allergic to several of the usual party ingredients.

If she is attending a party at someone else's house, ask the parent what will be served. If these foods are not included in your child's diet, *Substitute!* (This is the guide-word for parents of allergic children.)

Small gelatin cubes rolled in granulated sugar can substitute quite well for gum drops; a cupcake can be brought to take the place of birthday cake, and ice cream or ices can be brought from home, as can juice if necessary. With this out of the way, a child can concentrate on enjoying the rest of the party.

Several of the companies which produce milk-free formulas give out recipes for ice cream, but there are other, more tasty alternatives. If your child can tolerate corn, Mocha Mix frozen dessert (containing corn) is a delicious choice which comes in several flavors. If not, sorbets and ices are easy to make. (See Recipe section.)

"ICE CREAMS"

A. Contains soy and corn syrup
1 cup Dzertwhip®
1/2 cup sugar
1/8 teaspoon salt
Coffee Rich®
Balance of 2 cartons Dzertwhip® and enough Coffee Rich®
    to make 3 cups

Over low heat, warm 1 cup of Dzertwhip, salt and sugar, stirring until the sugar is dissolved. Chill. Add the rest of the ingredients and churn freeze. This can also be made in freezer trays if it is whipped when half frozen.

Variations: Add 2 ounces carob powder dissolved in Dzertwhip mixture or 2 teaspoons instant coffee or ripe fruit, lightly sugared and placed in the refrigerator until the sugar is dissolved.

B. Contains egg and nuts

4 ounces chocolate or milk free carob (or 2 ounces
    instant coffee)
5 egg yolks
1/2 cup sugar
1 cup crushed toasted almonds
1 whole egg
1/2 cup margarine
1 cup water

Melt the chocolate or carob over low heat. Beat yolks and sugar until lemon-colored. Put in double boiler with carob (chocolate) and stir for 4-5 mins. Remove from heat. Mix margarine and water in a blender and add this to the egg yolk/carob mixture. Add the almonds and whole egg and blend well. Pour into trays and freeze.

C. Contains coconut

Coconut for 4 cups coconut cream (You can buy frozen
    coconut cream at Oriental food stores, or use shred-
    ded coconut.)
Boiling water
1/2 cup sugar
1/8 teaspoon salt
1 1/2 teaspoons vanilla (or 2 teaspoons instant coffee
    or sugared fruit)

To make coconut cream: Open coconut and extract the meat. Pour boiling water (1/2 cup per coconut) over it and let it stand 20 minutes. Pass through a fine strainer. After several hours of refrigeration, it acquires the density of cream.

To make ice cream: Warm 1 cup coconut cream, and in it dissolve the sugar and salt. Chill. Add 3 cups coconut cream and vanilla. Churn freeze.

WATER ICES

"Water ices" or sorbets are made in several different ways. The simplest method is to shave ice and pour fruit syrup over it. It is sold like this in paper cups by vendors in Puerto Rico and New York City. Another recipe follows:

2 cups water
1 cup apricot or other juice
2 tablespoons gelatin*
1/2 cup sugar

Boil the water and sugar for 5 minutes to make a syrup. Cool and add juice in which the gelatin has been dissolved. Freeze in churn freezer or in trays (mixing frequently).
*Kosher (pareve) gelatin or agar-agar (sold in Oriental food stores) contain no animal products.

To make ice pops, any acceptable juice can be frozen in ice pop molds. These are available at most supermarkets or through Tupperware® dealers. The Tupperware® ice pop molds are the most tightly sealed (excellent for carrying) and the easiest to open without losing the contents.

For birthday parties at home, a rice flour cake or potato flour cake (best if eggs are permitted) works well. If you make a rice flour, eggless cake, it will be VERY fragile and must be handled using the utmost care. (See Recipe section.) Otherwise fancy cookies can be used. Rice flour cupcakes also work well for an allergic child. They are not very popular with other children, so I have at times baked two kinds, placing the rice cupcakes in the middle of a large plate and surrounding it with the others (with a small paper barrier around the rice cupcakes). Always mark the "special" cupcake.

In order to avoid cake altogether, serve an "ices cake" (ices pressed into a mold and frozen) or this fancy gelatin "cake."

GELATIN "CAKE"

1 3-ounce package each lime, red, purple gelatin (or 3 table-
    spoons each of plain gelatin and fruit syrup to color)
3 cups boiling water
1 1/2 cups cold water

1 3-ounce package lemon gelatin
1/4 cup sugar
1 cup boiling water
1/4 cup canned fruit juice
3 cups whipped non-dairy cream

Prepare each of the gelatin flavors separately, using 1 cup boiling water and 1/4 cup cold water for each. Pour into separate pans and chill at least 3 hours. Cut into 1/4 inch cubes and set a few aside to use as decoration.

Dissolve lemon gelatin and sugar in 1 cup boiling water and stir in juice. Chill until thickened. Blend whipped cream into lemon gelatin. Fold in the gelatin pieces (not the reserves) and place in a spring-form pan overnight. To remove, run a spatula around the edges of the pan and open. Garnish with reserved cubes.

After all this, remember – children come to a party for fun, so don't worry too much about the food. As long as your child is happy with the food, the others probably won't even notice!

Children's Favorites

TODDLER BURGERS

Ground meat (any tolerated: turkey, lamb, chicken,
    beef, pork, or veal)
2 slices of acceptable bread

Cut out circles in the bread with a cookie cutter. Make a small patty of the meat and broil. (The patty should be the same size as the bread circles). Place the meat between the bread circles and serve. The toddler will have a "burger" which is soft enough to chew and will fit his /her mouth.

TODDLER'S CASSEROLE

1 cup cooked rice
1 10-ounce package frozen peas and carrots
1 can pre-cooked soybeans or small pieces of cubed meat

Cook the peas and carrots in a small amount of water. Add the beans or meat and warm, then mix with the rice. This can be reheated in a microwave and is a good "feed yourself" meal. The small pieces offer a challenge to the toddler just learning to pick up objects with thumb and forefinger.

BEEF JERKY

Remove all visible fat from lean meat. If desired, sprinkle meat strips with a bit of salt. Dry very hard if you are planning to store it for a long time. Place in tight-closing jars, and store in a cool place. For drying instructions see Home Preparation of Food section.

TURKEY OR CHICKEN JERKY

Remove any fatty tissue from the meat. Slice very thin. This is done more easily if the meat is semi-frozen. Salt or seasoning may be added before drying. For long term storage, dry quite hard. Store in a tight-closing jar in a cool place. For drying instructions see Home Preparation of Food section.

PEANUT BUTTER-FRUIT SPREAD

2 cups peanut butter
1/4 cup honey
1/2 cup chopped pitted prunes, figs or raisins

Combine all ingredients in a bowl and mix until well blended. Store in refrigerator until needed. Makes approximately 8 sandwiches.

HIGH-NUTRITION PEANUT SPREAD

3/4 cups peanut butter
1/2 cup raisins
1/4 cup grated raw carrots

Mix peanut butter with raisins and grated carrots. Refrigerate until needed. (This can also be made in a blender by first chopping the carrots and then blending in the peanut butter and raisins.)

PEANUT BUTTER

1 cup roasted peanuts

Place peanuts in blender and process at high speed to desired consistency. Use a rubber spatula to keep the peanuts flowing into the blades, if necessary. Add salt to taste (usually a pinch).

NUT BUTTERS (Filbert, Almond, Pecan)

1 1/2 cups salted nuts (or roasted nuts plus 1/2 teaspoon salt)
2 tablespoons oil

Put oil into the blender and add the nuts. Process at high speed until desired consistency is reached. Use a rubber spatula to keep the nuts down near the blender blades.

SOY SPREAD I

1/4 cup soy oil
3/4 cups soy powder

Mix the two ingredients together until smooth. Season to taste with salt, vegetable salt, etc. To make the spread "chunky," add ground soy beans (toasted and salted).

SOY SPREAD II

1/2 cup cooked soybeans
1 tablespoon oil

Place oil and soybeans in a blender and process until desired consistency is reached. This can be made "crunchy" by addition of chopped roasted soybeans.

HIGH NUTRITION SOY SPREAD

3/4 cup cooked soybeans
2/3 cup raisins (or currants)
1/2 cup raw grated carrots

Blend the soybeans to a creamy consistency. Fold in the raisins (currants) and carrots until completely mixed. Refrigerate until needed.

APPLE LEATHER

Spread applesauce in 1/4 inch layer on a thick piece of plastic wrap about the size of the food-dryer tray. (See Home Preparation of Food .) Dry according to instructions for your food-dryer.

Addition of 1 teaspoon ascorbic acid per quart of applesauce will keep the leather from becoming too dark.

Variations: To basic apple leather you can add pureed prunes, plums, or berries for flavor.

APRICOT LEATHER

Fresh apricots
Sugar
Ascorbic acid powder

Wash and pit the apricots. Place in blender and puree. Weigh the pureed apricots. To each pound of fruit, add 1/3 to 1/2 cup of sugar, according to taste. Add ascorbic acid–1 teaspoon per quart of puree (this keeps it from discoloring, and adds Vitamin C).

Spread on plastic wrap and dry. The thicker it is spread, the longer it will take to dry, and the chewier it will be.

PEAR LEATHER

Puree the pears and spread 1/4 inch thick on plastic wrap placed on drying trays (if desired, some spice may be added, but it is not necessary). Dry. (For drying instructions see Home Preparation of Foods section.) Wrap in plastic wrap, and store in a cool place.

DRIED PEARS

Quarter and seed the pears. To keep from browning, sprinkle with ascorbic acid solution. For drying instructions see Home Preparation of Foods section.

DRIED APPLES

You can slice the apples almost any way, as long as they are fairly uniform and not more than about 1/4 of an inch thick. Place on dryer trays. As you cut them, placing them in an ascorbic acid solution will prevent browning. For drying instructions see Home Preparation of Food section.

DRIED BANANAS

Choose bananas which are fully ripe (skins should be completely spotted with brown). Slice in half, across, and then in quarters lengthwise, to form "sticks." Dry. (For drying instructions, see Home Preparation of Food section.) When dry, wrap tightly in plastic wrap and store in a cool, dry place.

CREAMY BANANA DESSERT I

4 ounces dried bananas
Water, to make 1 1/2 cups of fruit and liquid
1/4 cup honey
1/4 cup oil
1 teaspoon vanilla

In blender, puree all ingredients and freeze to a soft-freeze texture.

CREAMY BANANA DESSERT II

2 frozen bananas (freeze by removing peel and
    wrapping tightly in plastic wrap)
2 teaspoons powdered sugar
1 teaspoon vanilla

Place all ingredients in a blender and process until creamy. Serve immediately.

APPLE CANDY I

8 apples
1/2 cup water
4 envelopes gelatin
4 cups sugar
1 teaspoon vanilla
1/2 teaspoon rosewater (optional)
1 cup chopped nuts (optional)
Powdered sugar

Make applesauce of the apples and water. Measure out 1 cup of applesauce and stir in gelatin to dissolve. Put 1 1/2 cups of applesauce in a saucepan with the sugar and bring to a boil. Add 1 teaspoon vanilla to the applesauce-gelatin mixture and 1/2 teaspoon rosewater (optional) boil hard for 20 minutes, stirring often. powdered sugar. Remove from heat. Add vanilla nuts and rosewater. Pour into a "buttered" pan and cool for severl hours or overnight. Cut and roll in powdered sugar.

BARLEY SUGAR CANDY

2 pounds sugar
1 pint water
1 teaspoon lemon juice
5 drops lemon essence
Saffron powder (optional)

Dissolve sugar in water and continue boiling until it forms a syrup. When it reaches 312°F add both the lemon juice and essence. Keep boiling until it becomes golden. Add the saffron powder (a very little bit), stir, and pour onto an oiled board. When cool, cut into strips and bend into walking-stick shapes. Store in an airtight container.

CARROT CANDY

1 pound scraped and shredded carrots (about 3 1/2 cups)
1 cup sugar
1/2 teaspoon salt
1 pound honey
2/3 cup chopped, toasted almonds (other nuts or soy "nuts")
1 1/2 teaspoon ginger
1/2 tablespoon grated orange peel, if allowed

Combine the carrots, sugar, salt, and honey in a large pot. Cook over low heat, stirring, to 260°F. Stir in nuts, 1 3/8 teaspoon ginger and orange peel, and cook 1 minute longer. Turn out onto a cookie sheet coated with 1/4 cup sugar mixed with 1/8 teaspoon ginger. Sprinkle the top of the sheet of candy with the rest of the sugar-ginger mixture. Cut with a hot knife and cool.

RICE CANDY

Puffed rice
Small amount of oil
Peanuts
Pumpkin seeds
Sunflower seeds
Sesame seeds
Nut meats (any kind, optional)
Honey or pure maple syrup

Heat a heavy pan on medium heat. Add oil to barely coat bottom of pan. Add the peanuts and seeds, and roast lightly. Add the nut meats and rice. Remove from heat and add just enough honey or maple syrup to coat.

LOLLIPOPS I

2 cups sugar
1 cup light corn syrup
1/2 cup water
1 1/2 teaspoons peppermint extract

In a heavy 2 quart saucepan stir together sugar, syrup and water. Cook over medium heat, stirring constantly, until mixture boils. Continue cooking until temperature reaches 300°F. Cool slightly. Add flavoring. Place lollipop sticks 4 inches apart on greased foil. Drop candy mixture over one end of each stick to form a circle.

LOLLIPOPS II

3 cups sugar
1 teaspoon vanilla
1/4 cup water

Follow directions for Lollipops I.

MOLASSES TAFFY

1/2 cup blackstrap molasses
1/4 cup raw sugar syrup
1/2 cup sugar

29

1 teaspoon apple cider vinegar
1 tablespoon margarine

Place all ingredients in a heavy pot, and cook over medium
heat, stirring constantly, for 10 minutes (soft crack stage, or 290°F).
Pour out on a greased board to cool. When it is cool enough to
touch, butter your hands and pull. Cut into pieces and wrap.

SOY TOFFEE CANDY

2 1/4 cups sugar
1 teaspoon salt
1/2 cup water
1 1/4 cups margarine
2 cups roasted soy beans (soy nuts)
1 teaspoon vanilla

Over medium heat, cook the sugar, salt, water, vanilla and
margarine to 290°F on a candy thermometer. Stir the soy nuts
(roasted soy beans) into this mixture. Pour into a well greased pan
and cool. Cut into pieces.

SESAME SEED CANDY

1 cup honey
7 ounces (approximately 7/8 cup) sugar
6 teaspoons water
15 ounces sesame seeds

Bring the honey, sugar and water to a boil and then cook over
low heat without stirring. When it reaches the soft ball stage, stir
in the seeds and cook until the seeds begin to turn a light gold
color. Pour onto a wet board and cut. Allow to cool, then wrap.

MARSHMALLOWS I

2 tablespoons unflavored gelatin
1/2 cup cold water
2 cups sugar
3/4 cup boiling water
1/2 teaspoon salt
1 teaspoon vanilla
Powdered sugar

Soften gelatin in cold water 5 minutes. Dissolve by stirring over hot water. Combine sugar, salt and boiling water in a heavy pan and cook, stirring constantly, until sugar dissolves; then cook until it reaches 280°F. Add melted gelatin and vanilla. Stir and cool slightly. Pour syrup into mixer bowl and beat at low speed 3 minutes. Beat at medium speed for 10 minutes or until fluffy and cool. Sift powdered sugar into a pan and pour mixture into pan. Spread until smooth. Cool until set, and turn out onto a board dusted with powdered sugar. Cut into cubes and roll in sugar. *Note:* Fruit juices may be used in place of part of the water.

GELATIN CUBES I

1 3-ounce package gelatin*, any flavor
1 cup boiling water
3/4 cup cold water

Dissolve the gelatin in boiling water. Add cold water and pour into an 8 inch (or so) square pan. Chill until firm. Then cut into cubes. To remove from pan, dip quickly in warm water and invert onto a plate. For firmer cubes, reduce the cold water. For softer ones, increase to 1 cup. *Use Kosher gelatin if animal products are not allowed.

GELATIN CUBES II

3 ounces plain gelatin
Flavoring (either fruit concentrate or vanilla)
Sugar, to taste
1 cup boiling water
3/4 cups cold water

Dissolve the gelatin in boiling water. Add the cold water, concentrate, and sugar to taste. If allowed and desired, food coloring may be added. Proceed as for Gelatin Cubes I.

GELATIN SPAGHETTI

3 ounces any flavor gelatin (or plain gelatin and fruit
    concentrate)
1 cup boiling water
3/4 cup cold water

Dissolve the gelatin in boiling water. Add the cold water and pour into a dish. Chill until firm. Force the gelatin through a ricer or through a large strainer, and pile in dessert dishes.

GINGER FRUIT GELATIN

3 ounces raspberry or cherry gelatin (or plain gelatin and fruit concentrate)
1 cup boiling water
7 ounces ginger ale
1 teaspoon lemon juice, if allowed
1 cup drained diced pears

Dissolve the gelatin in boiling water. Add the ginger ale and lemon juice. Chill until thickened and add the pears. Chill until firm.

POPCORN BALLS

1 cup sorghum
1 cup brown sugar
1 small piece butter or margarine
Popped corn

Cook sorghum and sugar until hard ball stage when dripped in cold water. Add butter and pour over popcorn. Stir and make into balls. Peanuts or roasted soybeans may be added.

PRETZELS (Rice, Soy, Potato)

1/4 cup rice mix
1/4 cup soy flour
1/4 cup potato starch
1 teaspoon egg substitute
1/3 cup water
1 teaspoon oil
1/8 teaspoon salt

Mix ingredients thoroughly. Roll out by hand and then roll in salt. Bake at 350°F on a cookie sheet for 15 minutes or until light brown. They will be crisp when cool.

POPPED RICE

1 cup brown rice
Steamed oil for deep frying

Let the cooked rice dry in a low oven until hard. Heat the oil in a pot to 375°F. Put several tablespoons of rice in at a time and cook until puffed. Drain, salt and serve.

PUFFED RICE GRANOLA

1 cup chopped dates
2 tablespoons honey
2 tablespoons peanut butter or molasses
1 tablespoon margarine, soft
2 cups puffed brown rice cereal
1/2 cup soy nuts or sunflower seeds

Combine all ingredients in a mixing bowl. Be sure to chill until you wish to use. Instead of dates, 1 cup chopped raisins or currants may be used.

SWEET PUFFED RICE CAKES

3 1/2 cups puffed brown rice
4 teaspoons toasted sesame seeds (optional)
1/4 cup margarine
1/2 teaspoon vanilla
1 cup sugar

Mix sesame seeds and puffed rice, and spread in a pan. Warm in oven while melting margarine over medium heat. Add sugar and vanilla and stir until dissolved and thickened. Pour syrup over warmed rice mixture and press into a greased 8 x 12 inch cake pan. Cool and cut into squares.

***

Note: The following cookies are made with soy flour. These are solid enough to make really good teething cookies, and they dissolve well, providing some extra protein while making the usual teething-cookie mess.

***

CAROB SANDWICH COOKIES

1/2 cup margarine
3/4 cup brown sugar
1 egg (or egg substitute)
3/4 cup soy flour
1/2 cup Jolly Joan Rice Mix
1/2 teaspoon baking powder
1/2 teaspoon baking soda
1/4 teaspoon salt
1 1/2 teaspoons vanilla
3 tablespoons carob powder

Beat the margarine until fluffy. Add the sugar and continue beating. Blend in the rest of the ingredients. Roll out the cookie dough between two sheets of waxed paper. Cut into circles and bake at 350°F for 8 to 10 minutes. After they are cool, frost half with sugar and water paste (confectioner's sugar, if allowed, or if not, a sugar syrup, starch and milk paste). Place another round on top to form a sandwich.

SWEET POTATO COOKIES

1 cup packed brown sugar
1/4 cup margarine
1 1/4 cup mashed, cooked, sweet potato
1/4 teaspoon nutmeg
1 teaspoon vanilla
2 cups flour (or 3/4 cup rice mix, 3/4 cup potato starch,
    1/2 cup soy flour)
1/2 teaspoon baking powder
1/2 teaspoon cinnamon
1/2 teaspoon salt
2 eggs (or egg substitute)

2 cups quick cooking oats
1 cup raisins

Beat together margaine and sugar until light. Blend in sweet potato and eggs. Add combined flour, baking powder, vanilla, and spices. Mix. Stir in the oats and raisins. Drop by teaspoonfuls on greased cookie sheet and bake at 375°F for about 10 minutes or until lightly browned. Cool.

MOLDED COOKIES

1 1/2 cups flour (or 1/2 cup each potato starch, soy flour, rice mix)
1/2 teaspoon baking powder
1/4 teaspoon cream of tartar
1/2 cup shortening
1 cup sugar
1 teaspoon egg substitute
1 teaspoon vanilla
6 teaspoons water

Cream the shortening and add the sugar, beating until fluffy. Add the flour and all the other ingredients. Beat well. Shape the cookies with a cookie press and bake at 350°F for 10 minutes.

FRUIT TAPIOCA PUDDING

2 1/2 cups fruit puree or juice (any fruit allowed)
1/4 cup quick-cooking tapioca
Pinch of salt
1/3 to 1/2 cup sugar, to taste

Mix the juice, tapioca, sugar and salt. Let stand 5 minutes. Bring to a boil. Simmer, stirring, for 20 minutes and stir again. Cool and serve.

QUICK CARROT CORNSTARCH PUDDING

2 cups soy milk
1/4 cup carob powder
1/4 cup cornstarch
1 teaspoon instant coffee (optional)
1/4 cup water

1/4 cup honey
2 teaspoons vanilla

Heat the soy milk in a very large pot until it reaches a boil. Meanwhile, mix the carob, cornstarch, and coffee. Stir the water slowly into the carob mixture to make a smooth paste. Add the honey. Slowly add the mixture to the simmering soy milk and stir until thickened. Cook slowly over low heat for about 5 minutes. Let cool for a few minutes, then stir in the vanilla. Spoon into serving dishes and chill.

SALTED PUMPKIN OR SQUASH SEEDS

Seeds
Salt

Wash and drain pumpkin or squash seeds. Sprinkle lightly with salt and spread on a cookie sheet. Bake at low heat (250°F) until lightly browned.

PARTY APPLE JUICE

1 bottle apple juice, chilled
1/2 bottle carbonated water

Mix one part carbonated water to two parts apple juice and serve.

RECIPES

VEGETABLES AND NOODLES

Nutrient Saving Methods for Cooking Vegetables

A. Stir-frying

Stir-frying is a quick, nutrious method of preparing vegetables. Almost any vegetable can be cooked this way, following a set pattern:

Heat 2 tablespoons of flavorless oil.

Add bite-sized pieces of vegetable, the toughest ones first, and cook for 1 minute each, coating thoroughly with hot oil. Put aside, and stir-fry any meat you may wish to add.

Add 2 tablespoons stock or water, 1 teaspoon (optional) sugar. Cover and continue cooking until tender, but still crisp. Do not overcook.

If desired, add thickener (1 teaspoon cornstarch or arrowroot powder dissolved in 1/4 cup cold liquid). Stir until thickened (1 minute).

B. Steaming

Steaming the vegetables in a steamer or large sieve over boiling water is another way to cook them without losing too many nutrients.

If the diet is limited, some variety may be achieved by changing the shape or the texture of the vegetables while preparing. Carrots can be sliced round, diagonally, julienne, shredded (this last will require slightly less cooking time), or even pureed once they are cooked.

ASPARAGUS AND PEAS

1 cup asparagus, cut into 1-inch pieces
1 cup peas
Cream sauce (See Soya White Sauce on Page 96.)
Parsley or chives

Steam both the asparagus and peas. Prepare the cream sauce, and mix it into the vegetables. Sprinkle parsley and/or chives over the top, and serve.

STRING BEANS AND WATER CHESTNUTS

1 pound fresh string beans
1 can water chestnuts, sliced
1 1/2 teaspoons salt
1 teaspoon sugar
2 tablespoons oil
1/4 cup chicken stock
Starch for thickening (See Stir-Fried Broccoli on Page 43.)

Stir-fry. (See instructions on Page 37.)

HUMOUS

2 15-ounce cans garbanzo beans drained (or equivalent
    amount of garbanzos soaked and drained)
2 tablespoons oil
1 teaspoon salt
1 clove garlic
3 tablespoons lemon juice
2 tablespoons toasted sesame seeds
1 tablespoon chopped parsley

Combine all the ingredients except the parsley until smooth. Add the dried garbanzos. Serve as a spread or hors d'oeurve. Sprinkle with chopped parsley.

BOSTON BAKED BEANS

1 cup great northern beans, dried
2 medium onions, peeled
2 teaspoons salt (3 if not using salt pork)
3 cloves, stuck in the 2 onions
1/2 cup molasses
1 cup brown sugar
1 teaspoon dry mustard
1 teaspoon pepper
1/2 pound salt pork or 1/4 cup margarine

In a large pot, cover the beans with 1 inch of water and bring to a boil for two minutes and remove from heat for one hour. Bring to a boil again adding 1 onion and 1 teaspoon salt. Simmer, pot covered, for a half hour. Discard water and onion. Heat the oven to 250°F and place bean pot or casserole with other ingredients mixed in it. Bury the onion in the beans. Cut the margarine and push it well into the beans, too. Bake, covered for up to six hours, adding water if necessary.

Beans can be soaked, frozen on trays, and sealed in batches to be used later for baked beans.

BAKED BEAN SANDWICH SPREAD

1 cup baked beans
1 teaspoon lemon juice (or 1/4 teaspoon ascorbic acid)
1 tablespoon minced onion
1/8 teaspoon celery salt

Place in blender or processor and process until smooth.

REFRIED BEANS

6 tablespoons melted or liquid shortening
2 15-ounce cans of kidney beans
2 teaspoons garlic salt
4 teaspoons minced onion, dry

Heat shortening in a frying pan. Add the beans and mash. Cook, stirring until dry, then press flat with the back of a large spoon. Brown and turn. When browned on the second side, serve.

BAKED SOYBEANS

2 cups soybeans (dried)
1 teaspoon salt
1 onion, quartered
1/2 cup molasses
1/4 cup honey
1/2 teaspoon mustard powder
2 tablespoons oil
1/4 cup soy sauce or a bit more salt

Cover the dried beans with water and bring to a boil. Simmer for 4 or 5 minutes and let stand for an hour. Bring to a boil again and simmer until done (1 hour). Put the beans in an oven-proof pot at 300°F, burying the pieces of onion in among the beans, and thoroughly mixing in all ingredients. Bake covered for at least 6 hours, adding more water if needed.

TOFU WITH VEGETABLES

1 teaspoon vegetable oil
1/4 pound mushrooms, sliced
1 carrot, sliced
1 small onion, sliced
1 cup fresh mung bean sprouts
2 cloves garlic, crushed
1/2 teaspoon sea salt
1 cake tofu, cut in cubes
3 tablespoons soy sauce
2 tablespoons sesame tahini
1/2 teaspoon honey
1 tablespoon tomato paste
1/4 teaspoon freshly ground ginger

Heat the oil in a wok or heavy skillet. Add mushrooms, carrots and onion. Stir vigorously for 2 minutes. Add all of the remaining ingredients. Cover the pot and steam for 3 minutes. Serve hot.

SOYBEAN PANCAKES

1 1/2 cups cooked soybeans
1 tablespoon parsley
1/2 small onion (optional)
1 teaspoon sea salt
1/2 teaspoon celery seed
1 stalk celery
1 carrot, cleaned
2 tablespoons potato flour
Oil

In a blender, puree all the ingredients except the flour and the oil. With the blender going, add the potato flour, a bit at a time, and process until the mixture is smooth. Heat the oil in a heavy skillet and place the mixture by spoonfuls into the pan. Allow the mixture to become crisp on one side before turning. Serve warm.

STUFFED BEAN CURD

3 pieces of fresh Chinese bean curd
1/2 pound finely minced chicken
3 finely chopped scallions
2 1/2 teaspoons light oil
2 teaspoons soy sauce
1 1/2 teaspoon sherry or rice wine

Cut each bean curd into 2 triangular pieces. Very carefully slit one corner with a knife. Gently scoop out bean curd. Make a deep pocket. Combine minced chicken, scallions, 1 teaspoon oil, 1 teaspoon soy sauce and sherry. Mix very well. Gently spoon into bean curd. Place stuffed bean curds on an oven-proof plate. Cover with remaining oil and soy sauce. Place plate inside a steamer. Cover and steam 25 to 30 minutes.

STIR-FRIED SOY (BEAN) SPROUTS AND VEGETABLES

1 tablespoon oil
1 clove garlic, split
1 teaspoon sea salt
3 stalks bok choy, sliced (or celery)
2 tablespoons chopped green pepper
1 small onion, sliced
1/2 teaspoon grated fresh ginger
3 stalks celery
2 cups soybean sprouts
1 teaspoon arrowroot
1/2 cup water
1/2 cup tofu, diced
1 tablespoon soy sauce

Heat the oil in a large skillet or wok. Add the garlic. Brown garlic, then discard. Add the salt. Toss in the bok choy, onion, pepper and 3 stalks celery. Stir over high heat until the onion becomes translucent. Stir in the sprouts for about 1 minute. Mix the arrowroot with the water, add the mixture to the vegetables and bring rapidly to a boil, stirring. Stir in the soy sauce. Add the tofu and stir very gently, just to heat.

SOY BREAKFAST SAUSAGE

1/2 cup cornmeal
1/2 cup soy granules
1/2 cup buckwheat flour
1 1/2 teaspoons sage
1 1/2 teaspoons black pepper
1/4 teaspoon powdered garlic
3 cups of water

Mix dry ingredients with 1 cup of the water. Heat the remaining 2 cups of water to a boil, and gradually stir in the corn-soy mixture. Simmer over low heat, stirring, for about 10 minutes. Pour mixture into oiled loaf pan and chill thoroughly. To cook, slip the mixture from the mold and cut in 1/4-inch slices. Saute in a little oil over medium heat until brown and crisp on both sides.

FRIED BEAN CURD (TOFU)

Bean curd
Salt or soy sauce
Oil for frying

Place the bean curd between two plates overnight, with something heavy on the top plate. This will remove the water. Slice no more than 1/2 inch thick and sprinkle with salt or soy sauce. Deep fry until the pieces are golden brown (or dark brown if using soy sauce).

SALTED SOYBEANS

Soybeans
Water
Salt

Soak the beans overnight in lightly salted water. Spread the soybeans on a baking sheet and bake in 350°F oven for half an hour, stirring every so often. Add other seasoning if desired and permitted (i.e. garlic, onion, etc.)

BROCCOLI

1 bunch broccoli
3 tablespoons olive oil
2 cloves garlic thinly sliced
1/2 teaspoon salt
1/2 teaspoon black pepper

Wash broccoli well. Remove tough leaves and stems. Cut into small sections. Heat olive oil in frying pan. Saute garlic until brown. Add broccoli, salt and pepper. Cook about 5 minutes.

BROCCOLI WITH BAMBOO SHOOTS

1 head of broccoli
1 can sliced bamboo shoots
Salt
1/2 teaspoon sugar
Oil (4 tablespoons)

Slice the broccoli into thin pieces and drain the bamboo shoots. Heat the oil in a wok or pan, and add the broccoli, stirring constantly. Add the bamboo shoots and seasoning, heat through, serve. *Variation:* Eliminate the bamboo shoots and substitute parboiled cauliflower.

STIR-FRIED BROCCOLI

Large bunch fresh broccoli
2 tablespoons oil
1 teaspoon salt
1/2 teaspoon sugar
2 tablespoons chicken stock or water
1 teaspoon cornstarch or potato starch, dissolved in 1 table
  spoon chicken stock or water.

Wash, and cut broccoli into pieces, separate the stalks from the floweretts. Heat the oil in the wok (or pan) and add the stalks. Coat with the oil, and cook for 1 minute. Add the rest of the broccoli, salt and sugar and continue cooking for another minute. Add the stock and cover, cooking for 2 minutes more. Add the cornstarch mixture, stir to thicken, and serve. (This last step may be left out, if you do not wish to add any kind of starch.)

COOKED CABBAGE I

1 head of cabbage, finely sliced
Cream or soy sauce
Salt to taste

Put cabbage in pot with 3 cups of water. Cover and cook for 30 minutes until tender. Drain off the water and add cream or soy sauce to moisten. Season to taste.

COOKED CABBAGE II

1 head cabbage, shredded
1/2 cup soy cream
1/4 cup vinegar
1 tablespoon thickening agent (flour)
Salt and pepper to taste
3 tablespoons brown sugar

Put cabbage in pot with water to cover. Cook 30 minutes or until tender. Drain. Add 1/2 cup soy cream. Mix thickening agent with vinegar and add sugar. Season. Heat through and serve.

RED CABBAGE

1 head red cabbage
1 sliced onion
4 cooking apples
2 tablespoons lemon juice
1 or 2 tablespoons sugar, to taste
Salt and pepper
Oil to grease pan
3 tablespoons water
3 tablespoons vinegar

Wash, trim, and shred the cabbage. Place the cabbage and onions, alternately in an oiled baking dish and season. Add oil, water and vinegar, and bake at 350°F for 1 hour. Peel and slice the apples, and sprinkle with lemon juice. Add to the cabbage, sprinkle with sugar and bake for 1 more hour. Stir in oil and serve.

RED AND GREEN CABBAGE

2 heads red cabbage
1/2 head green cabbage
1 tablespoon onion, chopped
2 cooking apples
1 teaspoon salt
1 tablespoon margarine
1/4 cup boiling water
1 tablespoon brown sugar
1 tablespoon vinegar
1 teaspoon chopped chives

Shred and rinse cabbage. Drain. Saute onion, and combine with cabbage. Cook covered for about 10 minutes. Peel, core and slice apples. Add to mixture. Add salt, water and mix well. Simmer until cabbage is tender (1/2 hour). Add sugar and vinegar, and simmer for 5 minutes more. Add chives and serve.

CARROTS COOKED IN CIDER

2 cups carrots, sliced
1 tablespon margarine
1/4 cup apple cider
Salt and pepper to taste

Mix carrots, cider, salt, and pepper and cook, covered, over a low heat until the carrots are done. Add the margarine, and cook uncovered for the last few minutes, until the glaze thickens.

BAKED CARROTS

1 1/2 cups grated carrots
1 1/2 tablespoons margarine
1/2 teaspoons salt
1/2 teaspoons ginger
1/2 tablespoon brown sugar
Pepper to taste

Mix all ingredients well. Place in a casserole and bake in a 350°F oven for 30 minutes. Serve.

CARROT CROQUETTES

1 cup raw carrots, grated
3/4 cup raw potatoes, grated
3/4 cup onions, finely chopped
1 large clove garlic, minced
2 scallions, finely chopped
3/4 cup flour
1 1/2 teaspoons salt
1/4 teaspoon freshly ground black pepper
2 eggs, beaten (or egg substitute)
1/4 cup water
Oil for frying

Blend carrots, potatoes, onions, garlic and scallions well. Combine flour, salt, pepper, eggs and water. Add carrot mixture. Stir well. Drop carrot batter by tablespoons into hot oil. Fry until nicely browned. Drain on paper towels.

PUREED CARROTS

2 pounds carrots, peeled and cooked
4 tablespoons margarine
1/2 teaspoon salt
A pinch of nutmeg (optional)
1 teaspoon sugar

Whip the carrots until smooth. Add the remaining ingredients and whip until thoroughly blended. Serve.

HONEY-GLAZED CARROTS

2 1/2 cups carrots, sliced
2 tablespoons margarine
1/2 cup chicken broth
1/2 cup honey
Salt and pepper to taste

In a saucepan, cook the carrots in the broth and margarine for 5 minutes. Add the other ingredients, and cook uncovered until the carrots are done, stirring occasionally to coat the carrots.

BROWN SUGAR-GLAZED CARROTS

3 cups carrots, sliced or "julienned"
2 tablespoons margarine
1/3 cup brown sugar
1/2 cup water or broth
Salt and pepper to taste

Cook the carrots as in Honey-Glazed Carrots.

CARROTS IN POMEGRANATE GLAZE

7 or 8 carrots, sliced
1/2 cup pomegranate juice
3 tablespoons margarine
1 1/2 teaspoons potato starch flour
Honey to taste for sweetening (or sugar, if honey is not
    acceptable)

Cook the carrots in the margarine until they are tender. Mix together the potato starch, juice, and sweetener. When the sauce is mixed, add to the carrots and cook gently, until the carrots are glazed.

CAULIFLOWER WITH CRUMBS

1 head cauliflower
8 tablespoons margarine
1/2 cup fresh breadcrumbs

Remove all leaves and the tough part of the stem. Wash and cook either boiling in lightly salted water, or in a microwave. In a saucepan, melt the margarine over medium heat and add the crumbs. Saute until they are brown and pour the mixture over the cooked cauliflower. *Note:* This sauce is also good for varying the taste of broccoli, string beans, etc., (which becomes quite important when you have a narrow choice of foods).

PUREED CAULIFLOWER

1 head cauliflower
2 teaspoons lemon juice
5 tablespoons margarine
Salt and pepper to taste

47

Cook cauliflower in salted water until tender. Puree in blender or food processor with the lemon juice. Mix in margarine and seasonings. Serve.

SHAKER CORN PUFFS

1/2 cup corn meal
1/2 cup boiling water
1/2 teaspoon salt
2 egg whites, stiffly beaten

Mix together first three ingredients. Fold in the egg whites, and drop by spoonfuls on a greased baking sheet. Bake at 350°F until puffed and gold in color.

SAUTEED CUCUMBERS

(Or Zucchini or Crooknecked Yellow Squash)

3 or 4 cucumbers (or 5 small squash)
2 or 3 tablespoons margarine
1/2 teaspoon salt
Chopped parsley (1 tablespoon fresh)

Peel and cut cucumbers into thick slices (do not peel squash if it is young). Saute in margarine until tender, and add parsley and seasoning. Serve.

COOKED CUCUMBERS

4 medium-sized cucumbers
Water
Salt
1/4 cup margarine
Salt and pepper to taste
1/2 cup toasted bread crumbs

Boil the cucumbers in lightly salted water until they are tender. Drain off the water. Melt margarine over medium heat and add bread crumbs. Saute until crumbs are brown. Mix with cucumbers. *Note:* This recipe may be varied by substituting chopped parsley for the crumbs, or adding a small amount of chives.

KASHA (Buckwheat) I

2/3 cups buckwheat
1 teaspoon salt
4 tablespoons chicken fat, oil or margarine
Water to cover

Place the buckwheat in an ungreased frying pan and cook, stirring, until it is a pale golden color. Place in a casserole, season, stir in fat or margarine, and cover with boiling water. Bake in a 275°F oven for 2 1/2 hours or until done.

KASHA AND PEAS

1/2 cup kasha
1 10-ounce package of thawed, frozen peas
1 1/2 cups of water, boiling
2 tablespoons shortening
1/2 teaspoon salt
1/2 cup onion, chopped
1 can mushrooms (optional)
1/4 teaspoon coriander
1/2 cup bread crumbs
1 cup vegetable broth

Heat the kasha over direct heat, in the top of a double boiler. Add the water, shortening and salt, stirring. Stir in the onions and mushrooms and cook over water for a half hour. Put 1/3 of the mixture in the bottom of a greased casserole, and add 1/3 of the peas. Sprinkle with coriander and salt to taste. Continue to layer until all ingredients are used. Top with crumbs and dot with shortening. Pour broth over it, and bake, at 350°F, until top is browned.

LENTIL CROQUETTES

2 cups lentils
2 cloves garlic, minced (optional)
1 onion, finely chopped
2 tablespoons olive oil
Salt (to taste)
1/2 teaspoon freshly ground black pepper
1 1/2 teaspoon ground cumin
1 egg, well beaten or egg substitute
Oil for frying

Cover the lentils with water. Simmer, covered, for 20 minutes or until tender and water is absorbed. Gently saute garlic and onions in olive oil until soft but not brown. Stir in salt, pepper and cumin. Add this mixture to lentils and blend well. Cool. Mash or grind lentil mixture. Form into small croquettes. Dip into egg. Fry in hot oil until nicely browned on all sides. Drain on a paper towel and serve hot. *Note:* Croquettes can be frozen until ready to fry. Recipe makes 4 to 5 dozen small croquettes.

MUSHROOM GARNISH

1/2 pound mushrooms
2 shallots (or 1/2 medium onion) chopped
1 1/2 tablespoons margarine
1/2 teaspoon salt
Pepper to taste
Tiny bit of lemon juice

Finely chop the mushrooms. Heat the margarine in a frying pan and add mushrooms, chopped shallots and lemon juice. Cook over medium heat until liquid is gone. Add the salt and pepper.

CHICK PEAS AND RICE

2 cups dried chick peas, soaked
3 cups cooked rice
2 teaspoons salt
1/2 cup margarine or chicken fat
1/2 cup water
1/2 cup honey

Drain the chick peas, and combine with salt and fresh water. Cook over low heat, covered, until tender (about an hour and a half). Drain. Add the chick peas to the rice in a casserole and mix with the rest of the ingredients. Bake at 350°F for a half hour.

SNOW PEAS AND WATER CHESTNUTS

1 pound snow peas
1 can water chestnuts, sliced
1 teaspoon salt
1/2 teaspoon sugar
2 tablespoons oil

Stir-fry. (See instructions on Page 37.)

SNOW PEAS, BAMBOO SHOOTS AND MUSHROOMS

1/4 pound mushrooms, sliced (or 7 Chinese dried
    mushrooms, soaked)
1 pound fresh snow peas
1/2 cup canned bamboo shoots, sliced
1 1/2 teaspoons salt
1/2 teaspoon sugar
2 tablespoons oil

Stir-fry. (See instructions on Page 37.)

PUREED PEAS

3 10-ounce packages frozen peas (or equivalent fresh peas)
1 carrot
1 leek
1/2 cup water
3 tablespoons margarine
1/4 cup soy cream
1/4 teaspoon dried thyme (if allowed)
Salt and Pepper to taste

Cook peas, leek, carrot and water in a pan until the peas are done. Remove water, carrot and leek and puree the peas until smooth. Add margarine, soy cream, salt and pepper. Place in a baking dish and dot with butter. Bake until heated through (350°).

DANISH POTATOES

2 dozen new potatoes
1/2 cup sugar
4 ounces margarine

Cook the unpeeled potatoes in boiling water until done (about 15 minutes). Cool slightly and peel. Melt the margarine in one pot, and cook the sugar in another pot until it is light brown. Add the melted margarine to this, and stir in some of the potatoes, stirring so that they are thoroughly coated. Continue until all the potatoes are covered, and serve.

HASH BROWN POTATOES

1 1/2 pounds boiling potatoes
Shortening for frying
Salt and pepper to taste

Peel the potatoes, keeping them in a bowl of cold water to keep them from oxidizing. Pat them dry and grate. Remove the excess water, and heat the shortening. Drop the potatoes into the shortening with a ladle, fry at high heat for 3 minutes. Reduce heat to medium and continue frying until done.

POTATO KUGEL

6 medium potatoes, grated
1 onion, grated
2 eggs (or egg substitute)
1/4 cup matzoh meal (or potato starch or rice flour)
2 teaspoons baking powder
1 1/2 teaspoons salt
1/4 cup margarine
White pepper if allowed

Mix potatoes with onion and salt. Add the eggs, flour, and baking powder. Blend in the margarine. Pour into the cupcake tin and dot with margarine or chicken fat. Bake at 350°F until top is crisp and browned (this may also be baked in a casserole of course).

OVEN FRIED POTATOES

4 large baking potatoes
Salt to taste
4 tablespoons margarine or other shortening

Peel and cut the potatoes in half lengthwise. Cut into thick
slices. Put in boiling water to cover and cook for 2 or 3 minutes,
blanching. Heat the oven to 450°F and into this put the potatoes
in a greased pan. Salt to taste and roast for half an hour, turning
once.

POTATO AND MUSHROOM PIE

6 medium potatoes
1/4 cup butter
1 teaspoon salt
1/8 teaspoon pepper
1/3 cup hot milk (or non-dairy creamer)
1 pound mushrooms sliced
2 tablespoons margarine
3 tablespoons chopped parsley
Paprika

Peel and quarter the potatoes. Cover with water and cook 25
minutes. Drain well and mash. Add butter, salt, pepper and hot
milk. Continue beating until creamy. Melt margarine in frying
pan and add sliced mushrooms. Toss to coat with margarine.
Cook over low heat 3 more minutes. Lightly butter 9- inch pie
plate. Spoon mushrooms into center and surround with mashed
potatoes. Set pie plate in a larger pan that has been filled with 1
inch of hot water. Bake at 400°F for 12 minutes. Garnish gener-
ously with parsley and paprika.

PARSLEYED POTATOES

16 small new potatoes
4 cups boiling water
1 onion, chopped
3 tablespoons margarine
3 tablespoons parsley, chopped
Salt and pepper to taste

53

Wash potatoes well. Drop in boiling water containing onion. Cook, covered, about 25 minutes or until tender. Remove potatoes and peel. Gently saute potatoes in margarine. When well coated, sprinkle with salt, pepper and parsley. Serve hot.

POTATO PANCAKES

2 cups raw grated potatoes (finely grated)
2 eggs, beaten (or equivalent egg substitute)
1/2 teaspoon salt
1/2 teaspoon baking powder
2 tablespoons flour (rice or wheat etc. but not potato)
2 tablespoons grated onion (optional)
Oil or chicken fat for frying
1/4 cup margarine or shortening

Keep the potatoes in water to avoid oxidation while you are grating them. Drain and add all ingredients except the shortening. Mix. Heat the shortening in a large frying pan and drop in the potato mixture to form pancakes. Turn, finish cooking, and serve hot, with applesauce or sour cream (or sour cream) topping.

POMMES DE TERRE, PROVENÇAL

20 small new potatoes
3 tablespoons margarine
3 onions, finely chopped
3 tablespoons chopped parsley
Salt and pepper to taste

Scrub potatoes and boil with jackets on, in salted water, until tender. Peel skins carefully. Heat margarine in frying pan. Gently fry potatoes until golden brown. Remove to a warm serving dish. Add onions to margarine and fry until transparent but not brown. Return potatoes to pan. Cool 1 minute. Cover with parsley, salt and pepper. Serve hot.

CRANBERRY SWEET POTATOES I

6 sweet potatoes (or yams)
1 3/4 cups cranberries
1/2 cup margarine

2/3 cup brown sugar (light)
1 teaspoon salt

Cook the sweet potatoes, then peel and quarter. Place in a casserole. In a saucepan, melt the margarine, add the sugar, cranberries, and salt. When the berries have popped open, pour the mixture over the yams, and bake at 350°F for a half hour.

CRANBERRY SWEET POTATOES II

6 cleaned sweet potatoes
Margarine
2 cups whole cranberry sauce

Cook the potatoes in boiling, salted water and cover until tender. Drain and peel. Butter the baking dish and place halved potatoes in it. Spread the cranberry sauce over the potatoes and bake uncovered at 350°F for approximately 20 minutes.

RICE COOKED BY CHINESE METHOD

(For Crust)

Wash the rice under cold water until the water runs clear. This should be long-grain rice. Place rice in pot and fill to cover rice with 3/4" water. Bring to a boil over high heat, uncovered. Cover, and simmer on lowest heat for 15 minutes or until all the water disappears.

RICE AND APRICOTS

1 cup dried apricots, chopped
1/2 cup raisins
Boiling water
1 1/2 cups raw rice
3 cups chicken broth
3 tablespoons margarine
1 onion chopped
1/2 teaspoon curry powder
1/2 green pepper, chopped

Soak the apricots and raisins in water for half an hour. Cook the rice in the broth until done. In a frying pan, melt the margarine and saute the onions and pepper. Stir in the curry powder. Mix all ingredients and bake at 350°F in an uncovered casserole until done (about 30 minutes).

RICE AND BANANAS

1 cup rice
2 1/2 cups chicken broth
2 bananas, quartered lengthwise and chopped

Combine boiling chicken broth and rice in saucepan. Bring to a boil, and simmer until done. Add the banana pieces and toss. Serve.

RICE AND CURRANTS

3 tablespoons margarine
1 onion, chopped
3/4 cup currants, dried
1 1/3 cups raw rice
1 teaspoon salt (or less)
1/2 teaspoon curry powder
1/2 teaspoon saffron
3 1/2 cups chicken broth

Saute onion and currants in margarine until the onion is translucent. Add the rice and salt, and stir until the rice is coated. Add seasonings. Add the liquid, and bring to a boil. Reduce heat to a simmer and cook until all liquid is absorbed.

CURRIED RICE

2 tablespoons butter
1 cup rice
2 cups chicken broth
2 tablespoons curry powder
Salt

Melt butter in saucepan and add rice. Saute until golden brown and add broth. Bring to a boil and add curry. Cook over low heat until water is absorbed – about 20 minutes. Add salt to taste.

SAFFRON RICE (YELLOW RICE)

2 tablespoons oil
2 tablespoons onion (optional)
1 1/2 cups long grain rice
3 cups boiling water
1 teaspoon salt
1/8 teaspoon ground saffron

Heat the oil in a heavy pot which can be sealed tightly. Add the onions and saute until soft. Add the rice and coat well with the oil, stirring. Add the water, salt, and saffron. Reduce to low temperature, cover pot and simmer until liquid is absorbed (20 minutes). *Note:* Chicken stock may be used instead of water for a slightly richer flavor.

SIZZLING RICE

1 cup long grain rice
2 teaspoons salt
4 cups water
Oil

Combine all ingredients except oil in a saucepan and soak for 1/2 hour. Bring to a boil, cover, and cook for a 1/2 hour. Spread 3/4 inch thick on a greased cookie sheet or large baking pan and bake at 250°F for 8 hours or until dry. Turn to prevent burning. Break the now crusty rice into pieces, store (it may be frozen). To serve, heat oil for deep frying, and fry until golden. Pour into hot soup in a hot bowl.

This makes impressive noises when put into hot soup or covered with hot food!

FRUIT PILAF

1 cup long grain rice
5 1/2 tablespoons margarine or butter
2 cups boiling water
Salt
1/4 cup chopped dried apricots
1/4 cup diced pitted prunes

57

2 tablespoons slivered almonds (optional)
2 tablespoons each hot water and honey

Melt half the margarine and add the rice. Stir to coat. Add the water, and bring to a boil. Simmer for 20 minutes or until tender. In a frying pan, melt the rest of the margarine, and add fruit and nuts. Saute until slightly browned. Add the water and honey and cook until somewhat thickened. Pour the fruit over the rice in a bowl, and serve.

WILD RICE AND MUSHROOMS

1 cup wild rice
1 teaspoon salt
2 cups stock (chicken or other)
4 tablespoons margarine
2 tablespoons grated carrot
2 tablespoons diced celery
2 tablespoons chopped onion
1/2 pound chopped mushrooms
1/2 tablespoon chopped parsley
1/4 cup chopped pecans

In a large saucepan, melt half the margarine, and when the foam subsides, add the carrots, onions and celery, and saute until the onions are translucent. Add the rice and stir, coating thoroughly. Boil the stock and add to the rice. Bring to a boil and simmer over very low heat until the stock has been absorbed. In a small frying pan, melt the remaining margarine and saute the mushrooms and parsley. Add the pecans and cook for 2 minutes more. Combine with rice and serve.

SPINACH MUSHROOM RING

4 or 5 bunches of spinach, cooked, chopped and drained
Creamed mushrooms (See Soy Cream Soup on Page 108.)

Place the spinach into a greased ring mold, packed tightly. Place mold, open side up in a pan of hot water, cover, and bake in 350°F oven until thoroughly heated. Unmold on a large plate and place creamed mushrooms in the middle.

SPINACH WITH ROSEMARY

2 pounds spinach, washed and chopped
1 teaspoon rosemary
1 teaspoon chopped parsley
2 teaspoons chopped scallions
Salt and pepper to taste.

Place spinach and other ingredients in a pot. Cover and simmer for 10 minutes or until done. Serve.

HUBBARD SQUASH

4 pounds Hubbard squash
Salt and pepper to taste
1/2 cup brown sugar
Margarine

Bake squash in 300°F oven until tender (about 2 1/2 hours). Cut into serving portions and season. Add brown sugar, and dot with margarine. Place under broiler to brown, and serve.

SHAKER HUBBARD SQUASH

1 pound hubbard squash, cut into pieces
2 cups hot water
1/2 teaspoon salt
1/2 teaspoon pepper
3 tablespoons margarine
1/2 cup maple syrup

Steam the squash in the water and remove from shell. Puree and add margarine and seasonings. Mix well and serve. *Note:* Leftover squash may be used in place of pumpkin for pies.

Alternate method: omit water, and bake in 300°F oven until done, about 2 1/2 hours.

ZUCCHINI OR SUMMER SQUASH

Both of these may be cut and sauteed in margarine for a very fresh-tasting vegetable dish. Use salt and pepper to taste, but sparingly. If the squash is young, clean well, but do not peel.

ZUCCHINI AND APPLES

6 small zucchini, sliced
3 tart apples, peeled, cored and sliced
3/4 teaspoon coriander
2 tablespoons brown sugar
Salt
Lemon juice (1 lemon) or 1/4 cup cider vinegar
4 tablespoons melted margarine
1/2 cup cider, apple juice, or chicken broth

Combine the zucchini, apples, and seasoning, and place in a "buttered" casserole. Add the rest of the margarine, cut in small pieces. Pour the liquid over this, and bake, covered for 15 minutes at 350°F. Uncover and continue baking for about 15 minutes or until the vegetables are tender.

TORTILLA ESPANOLA

3/4 cup oil (olive, optional)
3 tablespoons oil
3 large potatoes, sliced thinly
1/2 cup chopped onions
5 eggs
1 teaspoon salt (or more to taste)

Heat the oil in a large skillet and add the potatoes. Sprinkle with salt and cook over medium heat for 10 minutes. Add the onions, and continue cooking until the potatoes are light brown and/or soft. Drain in a colander. Put the 3 tablespoons oil in the pan and heat. Beat the eggs gently and pour into pan. Stir in the vegetables, spreading evenly, and cook until the tortilla is firm. Turn (put a plate over the top of the frying pan, and invert carefully – slide omelet back into pan). Cook until second side is done.

NOODLES

NOODLES

3 eggs
2 tablespoons potato starch
3/4 cup water
1/4 teaspoon salt
Oil to coat pan

Mix egg, potato starch, water and salt. Oil the frying pan. Pour 1 tablespoon of the mixture at a time into the pan, swirling, to spread evenly. This large noodle can then be cut to the desired shape.

RICE, SPAGHETTI OR NOODLES II

1 cup rice flour
1 tablespoon oil
3/4 cup water
Oil to coat pan

Mix the first four ingredients, until they form a smooth batter (quantity of flour may vary). Oil an omelet-type pan and place over a pan of water. Using 4 tablespoons of batter coat pan evenly and place over a pan of water. Cover and steam for approximately four minutes. Loosen noodle, and roll up to remove. This can then be stuffed or sliced to make long, thin FUN.

MEATS

BEEF

BRAISED SHORT RIBS

5 pounds lean short ribs of beef
1/2 cup acceptable flour (not potato)
Salt and pepper
2 tablespoons shortening
1 cup chopped onion
1 cup diced carrot
1/2 tablespoon chopped garlic (optional)
1/8 teaspoon thyme
1 cup beef stock
1 bay leaf

Season and dredge the short ribs in the flour, preheat the oven to 500°F. Put the ribs in a shallow roasting pan and brown in the oven for 20 minutes. Melt the shortening in a heavy, large flameproof casserole. When the foam subsides, add the vegetables and thyme and cook until the vegetables are lightly browned. Add the browned ribs, the stock and bring to a boil. Add the bay leaf and cover. Reduce the oven heat to 325°F and braise for 1 hour until the meat is tender. Put the ribs on a plate, strain juice through a sieve, and skim the fat. Pour the juices over the meat, and serve.

PEPPER STEAK

1 flank steak, trimmed
2 large green peppers, seeded and cut into bite-sized pieces.
2 quarter-size slices of ginger-root, peeled
1 tablespoon rice wine or dry sherry (optional)
1 teaspoon sugar
1 tablespoon soy sauce
1/4 cup oil
Thickener, if desired

Freeze the flank steak, spread flat for 15 minutes or so, until it is more solid. This makes it easier to slice. Slice with a cleaver or very sharp knife, into thin diagonal slices, about 1 1/2 inches long. Mix the rice wine, sugar, soy sauce and starch, if used, in a bowl, and add the meat, coating thoroughly. In a wok or pot, heat 1 tablespoon oil, and add the pepper. Cook until tender. Add the rest of the oil, and stir in the ginger. Add the meat, and cook until done. Add peppers and heat.

BEEF-STUFFED CABBAGE

1 head cabbage
1 1/2 pounds ground beef
1 onion, grated
1/2 teaspoon salt
4 tablespoons brown sugar
4 tablespoons apple cider vinegar
1/4 cup raisins
2 cups water
3 beef bones
3 tablespoons uncooked rice
Oil

Saute the onion in a tiny bit of oil. Put aside. Simmer the beef bones in a large casserole, with the water, for 1/2 hour. Mix in a large bowl, the onion, meat, salt, and rice. In a large pot, soak the cabbage leaves in boiling water for 30 minutes, until pliable. Place the meat mixture in the middle of the leaves, rolling them over, and tucking in the ends. Place these bundles in the casserole, add the brown sugar, vinegar and raisins, and simmer for hours.

BEEF WITH GREEN BEANS

1/2 pound flank steak
1/2 pound Chinese long beans (or stringbeans)
Water
1/2 teaspoon sugar
1 tablespoon soy sauce
4 teaspoons oil
1 slice ginger root, size of a quarter
Chopped green onions

Combine the sugar and soy sauce. Add 1 tablespoon oil and the ginger root, and marinate the meat in this for 1 hour. Slice the beans diagonally, and cook in boiling water until tender, but crisp. Drain, saving 1/2 cup of the liquid. Heat the remaining oil in a wok or pan. Add the beans and stir-fry for 3 minutes. Remove. Add the beef and brown. Return the beans plus the marinade and bean-water, and heat through. Serve.

BEEF WITH CELLOPHANE NOODLES

4 ounces cellophane noodles
1 pound flank steak, cut in strings (julienne)
1 tablespoon soy sauce (or add salt)
1 teaspoon sugar
2 cups oil
2 green peppers, seeded and cut into pieces
Quarter-sized peeled pieces of ginger root
Pepper to taste
Thickening agent (potato or corn starch or arrowroot)

Heat the oil in a wok or deep fryer. Drop in cellophane noodles in small batches, allowing to puff up. Drain noodles, and pour off oil. Return 2 tablespoons oil to the pan, and when it is hot, add the green peppers. Stir-fry until it is tender, and crisp. Put aside. Add 2 tablespoons more oil, and when it is hot, the ginger root. Then add the meat and spice and cook until the beef has lost its pink color. Return the pepper to the wok, and heat through (remove the pieces of ginger). Serve the meat mixture surrounded by the noodles.

BOILED FLANKEN

4 pounds flank steak
2 tablespoons fat or margarine or oil
1 1/2 quarts boiling water
1 onion
2 carrots
3 stalks celery
2 springs parsley
2 teaspoons salt
4 peppercorns, if allowed

Brown meat in the fat or oil. Add the rest of the ingredients, and cover. Cook over low heat for 2 hours or until meat is tender. Strain the stock and serve as soup, or reserve for other cooking.

ROLLED FLANK STEAK

2 flanks steaks (large)
1 teaspoon thyme
1 teaspoon chopped garlic (optional)
1/2 cup wine vinegar
1 bunch fresh spinach
5 young carrots
1 medium onion, sliced
1/4 cup chopped parsley
1 teaspoon chili powder
2 teaspoons salt
3 cups stock
Water

Place the steaks, pounded flat, end to end. Pound the ends together. Sprinkle with the first three ingredients and cover the meat with spinach. Place the carrots at intervals across the meat (lengthwise) and cover evenly with the other ingredients (except stock). Roll and tie the roast. Place in a casserole and add the stock and water so the liquid comes half way up the roast. Cover and bake at 350°F for 1 hour. Allow to rest, and cut the string. Slice and serve.

HASH (Beef and Potatoes)

Bread crumbs for topping
2 cups leftover cooked beef
3 large potatoes, peeled
1/2 onion, chopped
3/4 teaspoon salt
1/4 teaspoon white pepper
2 cups meat juices and/or broth

Butter a casserole (margarine may be used). Grind or chop meat and potatoes. Add chopped onion and all other ingredients and mix thoroughly. Sprinkle with crumbs and bake in a 375°F oven until the crumbs are brown (45 minutes).

65

STUFFED CABBAGE

1 head cabbage
2 tablespoons fat or oil
1 1/2 onions, sliced
2 cups canned tomatoes (if tomatoes are not allowed, add this
    same amount of water, or add 1 cup water and 1 cup wine)
1/2 teaspoons salt
3 or 4 beef bones
1 pound ground beef
4 tablespoons uncooked rice
2 tablespoons grated onion or chopped celery
1 egg or egg substitute
3 tablespoons honey
1/4 cup lemon juice or 1 teaspoon ascorbic acid
1/4 cup seedless raisins

Soak the cabbage in boiling water 15 min. Remove 12 to 20 leaves of cabbage for stuffing. Heat the fat in a heavy saucepan, and brown onions. Add tomatoes, 1/2 of the salt and the beef bones, and simmer for a half hour. Mix the beef, rice, grated onion, egg, and bit of water, if necessary for moistness. Place mixture in the middle of leaves, fold over sides, and tuck in ends. Add the honey, lemon juice and raisins and cook over low heat for two hours.

CHUCK ROAST WITH CABBAGE

1 small head cabbage, cut in wedges
1 3 1/2 pound chuck roast
1 large onion, cut in quarters
4 large carrots, cut into large pieces
2 stalks of celery, cut
1 bay leaf
2 tablespoons vinegar
Salt
5 cups water
3 tablespoons margarine
Acceptable flour for thickener
1 1/2 cups beef broth (or juice from roast)

66

Season the meat, and brown. Place meat, vegetables, bay leaf, water and salt in pot and cook slowly until meat is tender. Remove the meat to a plate, turn the heat to medium-high, and cook cabbage. Cook for 20 minutes until done. In a saucepan, melt the margarine and add the flour. Add the broth and salt, and stir over low heat until thickened. Pour over meat and vegetables. Serve.

POTATO SAUSAGE

Casing (cellulose or animal)
1 1/2 pounds lean beef, boneless
1 pound lean turkey, veal or pork
6 medium potatoes
1 medium onion
1 tablespoon salt
1/4 teaspoon pepper
1 teaspoon allspice

Rinse and soak casings. Make sure that the meat is trimmed of fat, and grind together coarsely. Peel and chop up the potatoes, and mix all the ingredients thoroughly. Still using the coarse grinder, this time with the sausage stuffing attachment, fill the casing, dividing into the units desired. To cook, prick the casing and simmer, covered with water for half and hour. If you have frozen them, thaw before cooking.

SWEET-AND-SOUR POT ROAST

4 pounds brisket or chuck
2 tablespoons shortenings (oil)
2 onions, sliced
1 1/2 teaspoons salt
1 clove garlic, minced
2 black peppercorns
1 bay leaf
1 1/2 cups boiling water
5 tablespoons brown sugar
1/4 cup cider vinegar or lemon juice

Brown the meat in the shortening in a heavy pot. Remove the excess fat, and add all ingredients except the vinegar. Bring to a boil, reduce heat and simmer for 4 hours or until the meat is tender.

Add water, if needed during cooking. Add the brown sugar and vinegar, and cook for a half hour, stirring to prevent sticking. Remove the meat from the pot and slice, then replace. Reheat, and serve.

TZIMMES (Slow-cooked beef and vegetables)

1 pound brisket
1 teaspoon salt
1/2 teapoon pepper
2 cups water
1 onion, quartered
1 stalk celery, sliced
3 pounds sweet potatoes, peeled and diced
4 or 5 carrots, diced
1 1/2 cup brown sugar
(for variation, add 6 ounces prunes)

Season the meat with the salt and pepper. Brown the meat in the shortening in a heavy pot. Add the water, onion, and celery. Bring to a boil, reduce heat, and simmer for 3 hours until the meat is tender. Add more water if needed during cooking. Remove the onion. Add the sweet potatoes and carrots and cook for 10 minutes. Sprinkle with the brown sugar and then bake at 350°F for 45 minutes until vegetables are tender.

BEEF POT PIE

2 pound trimmed beef chuck, cubed
2 teaspoons salt and pepper
1/3 cup acceptable flour (not potato)
1/4 cup oil
1/2 cup onions, chopped
1 bay leaf
4 cups water
1 teaspoon chopped garlic
3 medium boiling potatoes, cubed
4 medium carrots, sliced
1/4 cup chopped parsley
Short crust pastry

Season the beef cubes with salt and pepper (if allowed) and

coat with flour. Heat the oil and brown the beef in it. Then remove the cubes to a plate, and add the onions and garlic to the oil, stirring until translucent. Add the water and bring to a boil, scraping the pan. Return the beef to the pan, add the bay leaf and simmer for 1 hour.

Roll a short crust pastry out quite thin, and place over the top of the casserole, cutting slits, and crimping the crust at the edges. Bake at 375°F (or if it contains soy and rice, at 350°F) for 45 minutes, until crust is done.

RICE NOODLE BEEF

1 1/4 pounds (approx.) rice noodles
1/2 pound lean beef, sliced thin
1/4 teaspoon sesame oil
1/2 teaspoon dark soy sauce (or salt)
1 quarter-sized slice of peeled ginger
1 clove garlic, crushed
1/2 pound bean sprouts
2 tablespoons oyster sauce, if permitted
Oil and salt

Marinate the beef in 1/4 teaspoon salt, soy sauce and sesame oil. Heat 2 tablespoons oil in a wok, and brown the noodles over medium heat on both sides. In another pan, brown the ginger and garlic in 1 tablespoon oil and discard. Stir fry the beef in this oil and add to noodles. Stir-fry the bean sprouts in clean oil and add, along with the oyster sauce and salt, to the beef-noodle mixture.

CHOPPED LIVER

1 pound calf's or beef liver
1 onion
1 hard-cooked egg (or 2 stalks sauteed celery to substitute)
3 tablespoons (approx.) oil
3/4 teaspoons salt

Wash the liver, and remove any membrane. Saute the onion. Then add liver and sautee. Grind or chop the onion, liver and eggs (or celery) and add spice to taste. A small amount of additional oil may make the mixture more moist.

69

VEAL

LEMON VEAL

1 1/2 pounds veal, sliced thin
Rice flour for breading (or wheat)
1 lemon, washed and sliced
1 1/2 cups chicken broth
1/4 cup sherry
Salt and white pepper to taste
1 tablespoon margarine (optional)

Cover the veal lightly with flour and brown in a large skillet. Add sherry and bring to a boil. Add broth and lemon and simmer until veal is tender. Remove veal and lemon slices and boil down the liquid to use as gravy. Add 1 tablespoon margarine.

VEAL WITH PEPPERS

2 pounds veal stew meat
2 green peppers
3/4 pound mushrooms sliced
1 1/2 cups chicken broth
1 onion, chopped
1/4 cup sherry
Olive oil
Salt to taste

Lightly coat the bottom of a large skillet with olive oil and brown the onions. Add the meat and brown. Add the rest of the ingredients and simmer until meat is tender. Serve.

VEAL RAGOUT

2 pounds cubed veal
3 tablespoons shortening
1/2 cup onions, chopped
2 tablespoons acceptable flour (not potato)
1 1/2 tablespoons caraway seeds
1 1/2 cups chicken stock (or beef)

1 cup mushrooms, sliced
Salt and pepper

Season the veal cubes with the salt and pepper. Melt the margarine, and when the foam subsides, add the onions and cook until transparent. Add the veal and sprinkle the flour and seeds over it, stirring to coat. Cover and cook over low heat, not letting the veal stick. Add the stock, bring to a boil and simmer until the veal is done (add the mushrooms with the stock). If it dries out, add more stock.

VEAL SPARERIBS

Breast of veal, bones cracked
1 onion, grated
1 tablespoon shortening
1 teaspoon garlic salt
1/2 teaspoon paprika
Acceptable barbeque sauce

Rub the meat with a mixture of garlic, salt, shortening, onion and paprika. Place on a rack in a large pan with water in the bottom of the pan and roast at 350°F for approximately 2 1/2 hours. Remove from the pan and cut the ribs apart. Brush with the sauce and place under broiler until crisp.

LAMB

CROWN OF LAMB

5 pounds of lamb (rib chops still joined and formed in a circle)
Water
Salt
Peas
Small roasting potatoes

Cover the tips of the bones with oiled parchment, and begin roasting in a 450°F oven. After 15 minutes, reduce heat to 350°F, season, and add peeled small potatoes. Roast for one hour, basting. Turn the potatoes a few times. Place on a dish, fill the crown with cooked peas, and surround with the potatoes.

CROWN ROAST OF LAMB

4 1/2 pounds crown roast
2 teaspoons salt
1 teaspoon pepper, if allowed
1 teaspoon rosemary
15 small new potatoes, peeled
3 cups cooked peas
2 tablespoons margarine

Season the chops with the spices, and cover the ends with foil to prevent burning. Place the roast on a rack in a roasting pan and surround the rack with the small peeled potatoes. Put this in a preheated 475°F oven and reduce the heat to 400°F. Baste the potatoes with the drippings from the roast, and cook for about 1 hour and a quarter, until done. Place on a platter, and fill the center with the peas, remove the foil, surround with the potatoes, and serve.

APRICOT BASTED LEG OF LAMB

As the leg of lamb roasts (in a slow oven), baste frequently with a mixture of 1 cup apricot puree, 1/3 cup sugar and 2 teaspoons lemon juice (or 1/4 teaspoon ascorbic acid).

LAMB AND CABBAGE

3 1/2 pounds breast of lamb
2 tablespoons oil
1/3 cup acceptable flour (rice)
1 1/2 pounds cabbage, cored and cut into wedges
1 cup celery, diced
1 cup onions, sliced
1 1/2 teaspoon salt
2 1/2 cups stock (any acceptable, except fish)
1 1/2 tablespoons peppercorns in a piece of cheesecloth

Cut the meat into cubes, and brown in the oil in a heavy pan. Remove the meat and place in a large bowl, and toss in the flour until the meat is evenly coated. In a heavy, tightly covered, pot, place layers of meat, cabbage, celery, onions, and salt lightly. Deglaze the pan and add the stock to it, scraping the cooked bits into the stock. Add this to the casserole, and add the peppercorns. Cook until the meat is tender (1 1/2 hours).

LAMB WITH CHESTNUTS

2 tablespoons oil
2 pounds lamb (neck is usually used)
1 medium onion, chopped
2 or 3 carrots, sliced
2 tablespoons chopped parsley
1/2 cup white wine (or water)
3/4 pound chestnuts
Salt and pepper

Brown the piece of lamb in the oil. Add the onions and carrots, and saute until glazed. Season, add the parsley, wine, and cover. Simmer until tender (about 2 hours). Slit the chestnuts and place in a cake pan with a small amount of water. Roast in the oven for 15 minutes and peel. Add to the lamb, and cook for a 1/2 hour.

CHOPPED LAMB WITH FRUIT

1 1/2 pounds ground lamb
2 apples (golden delicious)
1/2 cup raisins or currants
1 medium onion, sliced
1 tablespoon parsley, chopped
1/8 teaspoon garlic
1/4 teaspoon salt, or to taste
2 cups cabbage, shredded
Any acceptable thickener
Chicken broth
Rice, cooked

Cook the meat in a heavy skillet, stirring. Then remove, and saute the onion until translucent. Add the apples (they may be peeled, if desired) and raisins or currants, the parsley, garlic and salt. Simmer covered for about 10 minutes. Add the cabbage and cook for an additional five minutes. Using an acceptable thickener, add to either broth or water and mix into the pan. When thickened, serve over the rice.

LEMON LAMB

2 pounds cubed lamb
4 tablespoons oil
1 lemon, thinly sliced
1/2 teaspoon cinnamon
Pinch saffron
Salt and pepper
1 1/2 cups lamb stock

Brown the pieces of lamb in the oil. Cover with the lemon slices, and the cinnamon, and season to taste. Add the saffron to the stock, and this to the pan. Stir well, cover, and simmer until the lamb is tender (about an hour and 15 minutes).

LAMB AND LIMA BEAN STEW

2 1/2 cups lima beans
6 cups water
3 pounds lean lamb cut into cubes
1 1/2 teaspoons salt
1/4 cup acceptable flour (not potato)
1/4 cup oil
1 teaspoon chopped garlic
3 cups chicken stock
1 teaspoon dried oregano
1/4 teaspoon thyme
1/4 teaspoon rosemary
2 carrots, sliced
6 small boiling onions, peeled
3 stalks celery, sliced
1/4 pound mushrooms, stemmed
2 tablespoons shortening

Boil the 6 cups of water and add lima beans. Boil for 2 minutes and remove from heat. Allow to soak for 1 hour. Season the lamb cubes with salt and pepper and coat with flour, shaking off the excess. Heat the oil and brown the lamb cubes. Transfer to a plate and set aside. Pour off all but 2 tablespoons of the fat and saute the onions and garlic. Add the stock and bring to a boil, scraping in all the pan juices. Add the spices and simmer, covered, for a half hour more with the meat. Saute the mushrooms in the 2 table-spoons of shortening and add to the casserole. Cook for a few minutes more. Serve.

LAMB AND PEARS

2 tablespoons margarine
2 tablespoons oil
3 pounds boneless lean lamb in pieces
Salt
Pepper
2 pounds pear halves and liquid
1 tablespoon cider vinegar
1 tablespoon Worcestershire sauce (optional)
1 1/2 teaspoons brown sugar
1/2 teaspoon nutmeg
5 scallions, chopped
3 stalks celery, chopped

In a flameproof casserole, heat the oil and margarine and brown the lamb. Discard fat. Combine the spices, vinegar, worchestershire sauce, sugar, and pear liquid and stir. Return the lamb to the casserole and bake at 350°F for 1 1/2 hours, adding vegetables during the last 20 minutes and the pears for the last 10 minutes.

LAMB PIE WITH DILL

3 pounds stewing lamb (shoulder) cut into cubes
1 large sliced carrot
1 medium onion, diced
1/2 cup celery
1 tablespoon vinegar
1 teaspoon sugar
1/2 cup soy cream
2 egg yolks, or substitute
1 teaspoon dill
Piecrust or mashed potatoes for topping
Thickening agent

Place meat (salted to taste), carrot, onion, and celery in water to cover. Simmer 1 to 1 1/2 hours until meat is tender. Skim, then drain liquid into a saucepan and add allowed thickener. Add sugar

75

and vinegar. Beat the cream and egg yolks together and stir into the sauce. Put meat, sauce and dill in a pie dish and cover, either with crust or mashed potatoes. Bake in a 350°F oven until warmed through or until crust is crisp.

RICE WITH LAMB

1 pound cubed boneless lamb shoulder
1/4 cup oil
3 carrots, julienned
2 medium onions, chopped coarsely
3 cups long-grain white rice
2 teaspoons salt
1/2 teaspoon pepper
6 cups cold water

Heat the oil in the frying pan, and saute the lamb until evenly browned. Place lamb in a casserole. To the fat, add the carrots and 3 cups onions. Saute until the onions are clear. Add the rice, and stir until thoroughly coated. Combine the ingredients in the casserole, and add water. Bring to a boil, and reduce the heat. Simmer for 20 minutes, and season to taste. Serve.

BROILED LAMB SAUSAGE

2 pounds lean ground lamb
3 tablespoons mint leaves
1/4 cup chopped onions
2 teaspoons salt

Thoroughly combine all ingredients in a large bowl. Shape the meat mixture into sausage shapes and place on a broiler tray. Broil 4 inches away from the heat, turning until evenly done. Serve.

PORK

SHAKER SAUSAGE MEAT I

5 pounds fat pork meat
15 pounds lean pork
1/2 cup salt
1/2 tablespoon red pepper
1 1/2 tablespoons black pepper
2 1/2 tablespoons ground sage
1 tablespoon sugar

Run the meat through the meat chopper two times. Thoroughly mix all ingredients. Roll into a cylinder and wrap in cheesecloth. Refrigerate. To use, cut into slices and saute. Use within 2 weeks, or may be frozen if wrapped properly.

SHAKER SAUSAGE MEAT II

5 pounds lean pork tenderloin (boned)
5 pounds fat pork
4 tablespoons ground sage
1 tablespoon black pepper
1 1/2 teaspoons salt
1 teaspoon ground allspice
1 teaspoon ground cloves

Prepare as above.

CHICKEN

RICE CEREAL "FRIED CHICKEN"

6 chicken breasts or thighs (skin on or off)
1/3 cup Mocha Mix or other "milk"
1/2 cup crispy rice cereal
Vegetable oil (if chicken is without skin)

Coat chicken parts in Mocha Mix and crushed rice cereal. Place in a lightly oiled baking pan and bake at 350°F for a half hour or until done.

CHICKEN AND APPLES

2 tablespoons margarine
2 tablespoons oil
Chicken parts
Salt
Pepper (if allowed)
3 tablespoons allowed flour for roux
6 carrots, sliced
8 small onions
4 apples, peeled and sliced
1 8-ounce package frozen peas
3 cups chicken broth

Heat the oil in a flameproof casserole. Brown the chicken and season. Add 2 cups chicken broth, and the vegetables. Bake for a half hour at 350°F. Add the apple slices and continue cooking for 20 minutes. Add peas and cook for 10 minutes. Meanwhile, make roux. In a pot, melt the margarine and add an equal amount of allowed flour. Add the last cup of broth and stir until thick and smooth. Mix well with the broth in the casserole, and serve.

CHICKEN AND APRICOTS WITH CHINESE VEGETABLES

2 tablespoons margarine
2 tablespoons oil
Chicken parts
3 scallions, chopped
3 stalks celery, thinly sliced crosswise
Small can water chestnuts, sliced
1/2 cup chicken broth
Salt or soy sauce to taste
1/4 cup chopped, dried apricots
1/2 cup slivered almonds (optional)

In a flameproof casserole, heat the oil and margarine and brown the chicken. Remove chicken. Add the vegetables to the fat and stir-cook (5 minutes). Remove. Add broth and scrape casserole to deglaze. Replace the chicken, and bake at 350°F, covered for a half hour. Add the remaining ingredients, and continue to cook until the chicken is tender.

CHICKEN BALLS

Raw chicken breasts
Scallions, finely chopped
1 tablespoon sherry
1 teaspoon cornstarch, or potato or rice flour
1/4 teaspoon salt
3 teaspoons water
1 teaspoon peanut or other acceptable oil

Cut chicken meat into small pieces. Chop with scallions. Add sherry and salt. Blend cornstarch and water. Add to chicken mixture. Shape mixture into 1 inch balls. Heat oil in skillet. Fry chicken balls until golden brown. Drain on paper towels. Serve hot. *Note:* Chicken balls can be frozen until ready to fry.

APRICOT BARBECUED CHICKEN

1 pound apricots
3 tablespoons margarine
1 clove garlic
1 medium onion, chopped
1 frying chicken, cut in parts
1 tablespoon soy sauce (or salt)
1/4 teaspoon salt
1/4 cup packed brown sugar
1 teaspoon lemon juice (or cider vinegar)
1/4 teaspoon dry mustard

Pit one cup of the apricots and puree. Saute the onion, and the crushed garlic clove until the onion is transparent. Add the apricot puree, brown sugar, soy sauce, salt, lemon juice, and mustard to the sauteed onions and simmer. Cut the remaining apricots in half and place on chicken parts when one side has been broiled. Baste the chicken with the liquid mixture until done.

CHICKEN CONGEE I

2 cups cooked chicken, cut into chunks
1/2 cup long grain rice
4 tablespoons glutinous rice
4 quarts stock
3 teaspoons salt
1 1/2 cups lettuce, shredded

Bring the stock to a boil, and stir in the mixture of long grain and glutinous rice. Partially cover the pot, and simmer over low heat for 2 hours. Add the chicken and salt, and cook until heated through. Put on a platter and garnish with the shredded lettuce.

CHICKEN CONGEE II

2/3 cup short grain rice
6 cups chicken stock or water
2 chicken breasts, bones, and sliced thin
1/2 teaspoon salt
4 tablespoons water

Place the rice and 6 cups stock in a heavy pot, and bring to a boil. Reduce heat and simmer at lowest heat until done (about 2 hours). Flatten the sliced chicken by pounding thin, and add the salt and 4 tablespoons water. When the rice is done, remove from heat and add the chicken to it. Cover and allow to stand for several minutes. Serve.

CHICKEN WITH BEAN SPROUTS

2 chicken breasts, meat removed and sliced very thin
1 teaspoon salt
1 teaspoon rice wine or dry sherry (or water)
2 cups bean sprouts (fresh)
1/3 cup oil

Marinate the chicken in the wine. Rinse the bean sprouts, and discard those which float to the top. Drain and dry. Heat 1 tablespoon oil in a wok or large, heated skillet. When hot, add the sprouts and 1 teaspoon salt, and stir fry until tender, but still crisp. Remove from the oil. Put the rest of the oil into the wok, and when hot, add the chicken and cook until it becomes white in color. Add the rest of the salt. Return the sprouts to the pan and heat through. Serve.

CHICKEN FRICASSEE

1 3-4 pound roasting chicken
Rice flour with salt added
3 tablespoons oil
3 cups boiling water
1 bay leaf
1 teaspoon tarragon
1/3 cup parsley, chopped
1/2 medium onion, chopped
1 teaspoon salt
1 teaspoon pepper (if allowed)
1 cup medium cream or soy cream

Cut the chicken into serving pieces. Wash and pat dry. Coat with the flour mixture and brown in the oil. When browned, add water (to cover chicken) and all ingredients except the cream. Cover and simmer for 1 1/2 hours. The rice flour coating will have thickened the broth. Remove the chicken and place on a platter. Add the cream to the pot and simmer, stirring, until the sauce is done (slightly thickened). Pour over chicken, and serve.

POTATO STARCH FRIED CHICKEN

1 package chicken parts
Pepper to taste
1 teaspoon soy sauce
1/8 teaspoon ginger
1/8 teaspoon white pepper, if allowed
2 teaspoons sherry or rice wine
1 teaspooon sesame oil
1/2 teaspoon salt

Coating:
1/3 cup potato starch
5 1/2 teaspoons water
1/8 teaspoon salt

Dip:
1/4 cup jellied cranberry sauce melted with 1/8 teaspoon salt

Remove bones and skin from chicken, and cut into large bite-size pieces. Marinate these in a blend of the rice wine, sesame oil, ginger, pepper, soy sauce and salt. Coat the pieces of chicken with a thin layer of mixture and deep fry in 350°F oil. Serve with the dip.

CHICKEN WITH GRAPES AND MUSHROOMS

12 half-chicken breasts, boned
3/4 cup margarine
1/2 pound mushrooms, sliced
1/3 cup rice flour (or any but potato)
2 teaspoons sugar
1/4 cup lemon juice
2 cups Thompson grapes (green seedless)
1 quart chicken broth
1/2 medium onion, chopped
Paprika (about 1 teaspoon)
Salt to taste

Wash grapes, and remove all stems. Sprinkle the chicken with salt and paprika to taste. Melt 1/2 cup of the margarine in a large frying pan, and brown the chicken. Put aside. Melt the rest of the margarine, and saute the mushrooms and onion. Add the sugar and the flour and stir. Add chicken and lemon juice, and the broth. Simmer for a half hour, until done. Add the grapes for the last few minutes. Season to taste, and serve.

CHICKEN HASH

1 medium onion, chopped
1/4 cup margarine
4 small potatoes, cooked and chopped
2 1/2 cups cooked chicken, chopped
1/2 cup chicken stock
1/3 to 1/2 cup soy cream for moistening
1/4 cup chopped parsley
Salt and pepper

Saute the onion in pan until clear. Add potatoes, salt, pepper and saute. Add chicken and stock, mix and cook over low heat for a few minutes, then add the soy cream and cook until brown. Add parsley and serve.

CHINESE CHICKEN SALAD

Marinade:
1/4 cup soy sauce
1 tablespoon brown sugar
1 clove garlic, minced
Dash pepper (optional)
1 cup chicken broth
3 chicken breasts, boned and sliced
1 medium onion, sliced
2 medium carrots, sliced
2 cups bean sprouts, washed
1/2 bunch scallions, cut to 6 inches and sliced lengthwise
1 pound spinach, washed and trimmed
1/2 cup almonds, sliced and toasted (optional)
Salad oil
Cooked rice

Marinate the chicken. Heat the wok, and add 1 tablespoon oil. Cook the chicken until white. Remove. Cook the onion for 1 minute. Mix in the carrots, green onion, and stir fry. Add the broth and return chicken to wok. Cook for about 4 minutes. Uncover and add spinach and bean sprouts. Cook for 1 more minute, covered. Stir. Remove to a platter and serve.

LEMON BROILED CHICKEN

Parts of 2 chickens
1/2 cup lemon juice
1 tablespoon lemon peel
1 teaspoon salt
1 onion, minced
1/4 cup melted margarine or butter
Pinch of saffron in 1 tablespoon hot water

Make marinade of the lemon juice, lemon peel, salt and onion. Place the chicken in this and allow to sit for 1 1/2 hours. Broil, basting frequently with the marinade, until done.

CHICKEN LIVER AND APPLES I

1/2 pound chicken liver, cleaned
Flour (except potato)
1 thinly sliced onion
2 thinly sliced apples
1 tablespoon sugar
Salt and pepper
1 tablespoon sherry
4 tablespoons margarine

Coat liver in flour. Heat 2 skillets with 2 tablespoons margarine in each. In first skillet, saute onions, then liver. In the other one, saute apples with sugar until golden and soft. Spoon apple mixture onto four warmed appetizer plates. Top with onions and liver. Salt and pepper to taste. Keep warm in oven. Add sherry to drippings. Bring to a boil. Pour over liver and serve immediately.

CHICKEN LIVER AND APPLES II

8 tablespoons margarine
6 apples, peeled, cored, and sliced
3 tablespoons sugar (optional)
1 1/2 pounds chicken liver, cleaned
Salt
1/2 cup cider
1 1/2 tablespoons lemon juice
Any acceptable thickener

Melt 4 tablespoons margarine, add apples slices and sprinkle with sugar, if desired. Cook until tender, but retaining shape. In second frying pan, melt 4 tablespoons margarine and cook liver for 5 minutes, stirring often. Add water and continue cooking for 5 minutes. In a saucepan, combine thickening agent, apple juice and lemon juice, cooking until thickened. Arrange apple slices on plate, add liver, and cover with sauce.

CHOPPED CHICKEN LIVER

1 pound chicken liver (very fresh)
4 tablespoons rendered chicken fat (or allowed vegetable oil)
1 large onion (red onion is milder)
2 hard-boiled eggs (to avoid eggs, 2 stalks of sauteed celery
    will lighten the mixture, or 1/2 cup of bread crumbs may be
    used if wheat is tolerated)
3/4 teaspoon salt
Pepper to taste, if allowed

Wash and clean liver very well. Drain. Saute the onions in 2 tablespoons of the fat; then remove. Cook the livers in the remaining fat until done. The liver may be ground or chopped with the onions, and then mixed with the other ingredients. *Note:* Chicken liver is milder than beef or calf liver.

CHICKEN MOLD

2 frying chickens
4 cups boiling water
4 tablespoons margarine
1 teaspoon salt
1 teaspoon pepper
1 teaspoon nutmeg, if allowed

Boil the chickens in water until they are tender. Remove the bones and skin, and chop the meat finely. Add the shortening to the stock, and reserve. Season to taste. Put chicken, and enough of the broth to moisten, in a loaf pan. Chill well. When it is cold, turn out of the mold, and slice.

CHICKEN MEDALLIONS

4 chicken breasts, boned
15 water chestnuts
1 scallion (optional)
Dash garlic powder
1 teaspoon sugar
1/2 teaspoon sherry, if allowed

1/2 teaspoon salt
3/4 pound snow peas, stemmed and cleaned
1 red bell pepper, or green if red aren't available
4 tablespoons oil for stir-frying
Sauce:
1/2 cup chicken stock
1/2 teaspoon vinegar (cider)
1 teaspoon sugar
1/4 teaspoon salt
Arrowroot powder (1 teaspoon) for thickening

In a food processor or blender, mince the chicken, water chestnuts and scallion. Mix with garlic powder, 1 teaspoon sugar, sherry, and 1/2 teaspoon salt. Roll mixture into small balls and flatten to make 50-cent-piece size pancakes. Stir-fry until lightly browned. Set aside. Stir-fry the snow peas for 1 minute. Set aside. Stir-fry the pepper for 1 minute. Set aside. Return all ingredients to wok and add arrowroot powder to sauce to thicken. Mix well and serve.

CHICKEN WITH PEARS AND VEGETABLES

2 tablespoon oil
Chicken breasts sliced in the Chinese manner (2 whole
    chicken breasts)
1 cup strong chicken broth
1 small can water chestnuts, drained and sliced
1 package thawed frozen peas
4 diced ripe pears
4 teaspoons soy sauce or salt to taste
5 scallions, sliced

Heat the oil in a wok or large frying pan and stir-fry the chicken until white. Add the vegetables and broth and cook for 2 minutes. Then add the pears and thickening agent, if desired.

CHICKEN PILAF WITH SOUR CHERRIES

2 pounds water packed sour cherries
Sugar (if desired)
2 tablespoons margarine
2 tablespoons oil

Chicken parts
1 onion, chopped
Salt
1 cup raw rice
1/2 teaspoon ground coriander
1 teaspoon cumin
2 cups chicken broth

Drain the cherries and reserve the liquid. If adding sugar, combine with cherries and simmer until dissolved (about 1/4 cup). Brown the chicken in a flameproof casserole in the oil and margarine. Season, and remove. Saute the onions in the remaining fat and add the rice and seasoning, stirring to coat each grain thoroughly. Combine broth with cherry juice to make 2 1/2 cups and pour over contents of the casserole. Bake covered for 1 hour at 350°F or until liquid is absorbed. Add the cherries for the final 15 minutes.

SHAKER CHICKEN PUDDING

3 1/2-4 pound chicken
1/2 cup chopped onions
1/2 cup chopped celery
1/2 cup peeled cored apples
3 tablespoons margarine or butter
1/2 cup cider
Salt and pepper
Nutmeg (pinch, if permitted)
Roux (made from 2 tablespoons margarine and
    2 tablespoons rice flour)
1 cup cream or soy cream
1 cup dry bread crumbs

Cook the chicken in water to cover. Remove the skin, bones, and meat, and set the meat aside. Saute the onions, apples and celery until tender. Add the seasonings and cider and continue cooking until the vegetables are soft. Simmer until the mixture is thickened. In a baking dish, combine all the cooked ingredients. Add to this the roux mixed with cream. Mix well. Top with the bread crumbs and bake at 350°F for a half hour.

ROCK CORNISH HENS IN TARRAGON SAUCE

2 game hens, split in half
Clove garlic
Salt and pepper to taste
1/4 cup butter
1 tablespoon tarragon

Preheat oven to 350°F. Prepare hens by trimming off excess fat at neck and tail. Rub well with garlic clove. Sprinkle with salt and pepper. Place breast side down in lightly buttered baking dish. Melt butter in small saucepan. Add tarragon. Mix well. Baste hens well with tarragon butter. Roast 1 hour. Baste every 15 minutes. Oven temperature may have to be raised to 450°F for an additional 10 minutes if hens are not golden brown in 1 hour.

TURKEY

HICKORY SMOKED TURKEY

1 turkey, fresh – no additives
Aluminum foil (if your grill is not covered)
Hickory flakes (2 ounce package)
Charcoal

Every half hour, sprinkle 1/2 cup hickory flakes (pre-moistened) over the coals. A 10-pound turkey will take about 4 hours, depending on the heat of the coals. If your barbeque is not a covered one, place a cover of aluminum foil over it to keep the smoke in. Baste the turkey occasionally. When the thermometer placed in the turkey breast registers 185°F, it is done. For extra flavor, coat turkey with marinade before cooking. (See marinade recipe below.)

Turkey Barbeque Marinade

1 pint sauterne wine
6 ounces soy sauce
1/2 cup salad oil

1 chopped onion
1 teaspoon garlic powder
1 inch-long piece of ginger root

PINEAPPLE TURKEY

1 pound turkey breast steak, cut in cubes
1 tablespoon cornstarch or rice flour
1 teaspoon salt
2 teaspoons cold water or chicken broth
1 teaspoon soy sauce (or a pinch more salt)
4 tablespoons pineapple juice
1 8-ounce can cubed pineapple
1 medium onion, sliced
3 tablespoons oil
1 cup celery, sliced
10 water chestnuts, sliced

Dredge the turkey cubes in mixture of water, starch, salt and soy sauce. Saute the onions in 1 tablespoon oil, and add celery and water chestnuts. Cook 2 minutes. Remove from the pan. Saute the turkey in the remaining oil until brown. Add the vegetables, pineapple and juice. Simmer until thoroughly heated. Serve with hot rice.

TURKEY WITH PRUNE AND APPLE STUFFING

12 pound turkey
2 teaspoons salt
1/4 teaspoon pepper
1 pound pitted prunes
1 cup water
4 cups sliced apples
1 cup dry bread crumbs
2 teaspoons lemon juice
1 tablespoon sugar
1/2 teaspoon cinnamon, if allowed

Season the turkey with the salt and pepper. Simmer the prunes in the water for 10 minutes, and drain. Add the apples, crumbs, juice, sugar and cinnamon. Mix thoroughly, and stuff turkey. Close the opening, and roast in a 350°F oven for 4 hours, or until turkey is done.

TURKEY STUFFED CABBAGE

1 pound ground turkey
Cabbage leaves
1/2 teaspoon salt
2 tablespoons uncooked rice
3 tablespoons brown sugar
3 tablespoons cider vinegar
1/4 cup raisins or currants
2 cups chicken broth (or 2 cups water, and 6 chicken legs,
    simmered for 1/2 hour)
1/2 onion, grated or 1/4 cup diced carrot

Saute the onion in a tiny bit of oil. Put aside. In a large bowl, mix the ground meat, onion, salt, and rice. Place this mixture in the center of the cabbage leaves, whick have been soaked in boiling water until pliable (30 minutes). Place the bundles in the large pot with the liquid, brown sugar, vinegar, and raisins, and simmer for 2 hours. If it becomes dry, add more liquid during cooking.

BAKED TURKEY-HAM SLICES

Turkey-ham
1/2 teaspoon cloves
1 or 2 apples
1/4 cup brown sugar

Slice turkey-ham in 1/2 inch slices and place in baking dish. Sprinkle with cloves, if allowed. Place sliced apple on top to cover meat. Sprinkle with brown sugar. Bake in a 350°F oven for 40 minutes.

TURKEY CAKES

2 cups ground cold cooked turkey
1/2 teaspoon salt
1/8 teaspoon white pepper
2 beaten eggs (or egg substitute)
1 tablespoon rice flour

1 tablespoon milk or non-dairy creamer
4 tablespoons melted butter or margarine

Combine in a bowl the meat, salt, pepper, egg, (or egg substitute), flour, and milk. Form into patties, and fry in the butter or margarine. Serve with sauce, below.

Sauce: To a standard white sauce, add 1/2 cup cooked celery, and chives to taste.

MEAT TURNOVERS

BLINTZES

2 eggs
1 1/2 cup water
1/4 teaspoon salt
3/4 cup flour
Margarine

Mix all ingredients until smooth. Allow to stand for 15 minutes. Coat a skillet with margarine and pour in a small amount of batter, turning pan so that the pancake is thin. Heat on low flame until it begins to loosen at the edges. Turn out onto plate and put the filling into the cooked side, in the middle. Fold up the edges to form a closed package, and saute in more margarine until browned on all sides.

Fillings:
2 pounds leftover beef
1 medium red onion, finely chopped
Salt and pepper
Shortening — to bind mixture together

Variations: Use standard dairy filling, or instead of filling, cover with a thin layer of jam and roll up.

KNISHES

1/2 cup flour
2 tablespoons vegetable oil
3 tablespoons water
Pinch of salt

Mix half the flour with the oil. Add water and salt and mix until it forms a dough. Knead, working in remaining flour, until dough is smooth and elastic. Cover and chill for 1 hour. Pull into rectangle which is as thin as possible. Cut out circles and place 1 tablespoon filling in the center. Fold in at edges and seal. Bake on a cookie sheet at 350°F for 45 minutes or until browned.

Fillings:

Potato
1 cup mashed potatoes
1/2 onion, finely chopped (optional)
3 tablespoons shortening
1 egg yolk (optional)
1/2 teaspoon salt
1/4 teaspoon pepper

Saute onion in shortening, and mix all ingredients. Place in center of dough circle.

Chicken
1/4 cup chicken broth or gravy
2 slices bread or matzoh, crumbled
1 cup finely chopped chicken (cooked)

Combine all ingredients, and place in dough.

Beef
See filling for Blintzes.

EMPANADAS (Turnovers)

1/2 pound lean ground beef
1/2 cup chopped onions
1/2 cup water
2 tablespoons raisins or currants
3/4 teaspoons chili powder
1/2 teaspoon paprika
1/4 teaspoon ground cumin
1/2 teaspoon salt
1 tablespoon oil
Double batch of acceptable pastry dough

In a large frying pan, combine the water, onions and oil, and boil until the water is gone. Add the meat, and brown. Stir in the other ingredients and combine well. Put aside. Roll out the dough, and cut in circles. Put filling in the middle, fold over and seal the edges. Bake on an ungreased baking sheet until the pastry is lightly browned (350°F).

VARIED MEATS

MEATBALLS FOR SOUP

Meat (chicken, turkey, beef or veal)
Flour (wheat, cornstarch, potato starch or rice flour)
Salt
Parsley, if allowed
Margarine or oil

Finely chop one pound of meat. Add just enough flour so that it will hold the ball together, and blend in the salt and parsley. Form the mixture into balls, roll in a bit more of the flour, and saute in margarine or oil until golden. Serve in soup.

RICE MEATBALLS

3/4 cup glutinous rice
3/4 pound ground beef, lamb, or veal
1/2 teaspoon ground ginger

1 tablespoon soy sauce (or substitute salt)
1 tablespoon water
1 tablespoon broth or sherry, or rice wine
2 tablespoons chopped scallions
2 tablespoons corn or potato starch
1/2 teaspoon sesame oil

Soak ingredients for a half hour. Mix all other ingredients. Oil a steaming rack. Form the mixture into one inch balls, and roll in the rice. Place the balls on the oiled rack over boiling water and steam for 1 hour.

MEAT SAUCES

MUSHROOM SAUCE

5 tablespoons margarine
1/2 pound fresh mushrooms, sliced
3 tablespoons onions, chopped
2 tablespoons acceptable flour (not potato)
1 cup beef stock
Salt
1 tablespoon lemon juice
1 tablespoon chopped parsley

Heat half the margarine in a heavy pan. When the foam subsides, add the onions and mushrooms and saute for 5 minutes. Melt the rest of the margarine, and add the flour, stirring constantly. When blended, stir in the stock and simmer for 10 minutes. Add the juice and parsley, and add seasoning to taste.

TURKEY GRAVY

Giblets and neck
4 tablespoons cooking oil
2 cups chopped onions
2 cups chopped carrots
1/2 cup dry white wine (optional)
2 cups chicken stock
Salt to taste

1/2 teaspoon thyme
Acceptable thickener

Chop the giblets and neck into smaller pieces. Dry, brown in the oil and remove from pan. Add the vegetables to the pan and cook until tender, covered. Then uncover and brown. Remove 2 cups of the vegetables, add the giblets, wine, stock, and water if necessary, to cover by one inch. Add herbs and salt, and simmer for 3 hours. Strain and remove fat. To this mixture, you can add the degreased juice from the pan, and then thicken according to the agent used.

MUSTARD SPREAD

6 tablespoons dry mustard
1 teaspoon salt
2 tablespoons oil
2 teaspoons sugar
Vinegar

To the mustard add a little boiling water. Add the salt, and the oil in small amounts, stirring. Add the sugar. Cook over low heat until it thickens and add the vinegar to taste.

APPLE CATSUP

1 cup sugar
1 teaspoon pepper
1 teaspoon dry mustard
2 teaspoons cinnamon
1 teaspoon cloves
1 teaspoon salt
1 1/2 onions, chopped finely
2 cups cider vinegar
2 apples

Peel, core, and chop the apples. Stew in water until soft, and strain. Add the other ingredients and simmer for 1 hour. Place in sterilized jars and follow canning instructions.

HORSERADISH AND APPLESAUCE
(For Fish and Boiled Meat)

4 apples, peeled and grated
1/2 cup grated horseradish
1/4 cup oil
2 tablespoons cider vinegar
Sugar or honey (optional)

Combine all ingredients in bowl and serve.

SOYA WHITE SAUCE

2 tablespoons soy oil
4 tablespoons soya powder
1 cup water or stock
2 teaspoons liquid lecithin
Salt and pepper to taste

Heat the oil in a pot, and add the soya powder, mixing well. Add the stock, and bring to a boil. Simmer for 5 minutes, stirring constantly. Add the lecithin, and continue stirring until it thickens.

SEAFOOD

CRAB MOLD

1 1/2 pounds cooked crab meat, cut into pieces
2 cups water
1/4 cup shallots, chopped
2 cups watercress, packed
1/2 cup parsley, chopped
2 teaspoons tarragon
1 tablespoon + 1 teaspoon unflavored gelatin or agar-agar
3 tablespoons mayonnaise
1/2 cup celery
Lettuce leaves

Boil 1 1/2 cups of the water, and add to it the shallots and parsley, watercress and tarragon. Boil for 1 minute. Drain, and discard the water. Puree the solid boiled ingredients. To the remaining 1/2 cup of water, add the gelatin and allow to sit for 5 minutes. Then heat until the gelatin is dissolved. Allow to cool. Mix the mayonnaise, pureed herbs, and cooled, fluid gelatin. Add the crabmeat and celery, and pour into mold. Chill until set, remove from the mold and serve on lettuce leaves. Garnish with parsley.

CRABMEAT AND SOYBEAN CURD

3/4 pound crabmeat
2 pieces fresh bean curd
3 tablespoons oil
1 teaspoon chopped ginger
1 scallion
1 1/2 teaspoon salt
1/4 cup chicken stock, or water
1/8 teaspoon telicherry pepper, ground
Chicken mixture
Thickener (optional)

Dice the bean curd. Heat the oil in a wok or pan. Add the ginger and the scallion (chopped), stir, and add the bean curd, salt, and stock. Cover and cook for 2 minutes. Stir in the meat and pepper, and heat through. Add thickening agent, if desired, and stir until thickened. Serve.

FISH STICKS

3 fillets of sole or allowed white fish
3/4 cup rice flour
2 tablespoons salt
1/4 teaspoon pepper, if allowed
3 eggs, beaten (or egg substitute and water)
3/4 cup dry bread crumbs
Oil or fat for deep frying

Cut the fish into one-inch strips. Mix the flour with salt and pepper, and shake with the fish strips in a bag, to coat. Dip the fish strips in the egg mixture, and then in the bread crumbs. Heat the fat in a fryer or deep pot, and fry the sticks until browned.

SALMON PASTRY

Any acceptable pastry, made with 4 cups baking flour
1/2 pound salmon, fresh
1 cup shredded carrots
1/2 cup chopped celery
1 cup chopped onions
2 black peppercorns
1/4 pound margarine
1/2 pound sliced mushrooms
1 tablespoon lemon juice
1 cup chopped onions
1/2 cup long-grain rice
1 cup chicken stock
1/3 cup fresh dill leaves
2 hard boiled eggs (optional) or substitute tofu
Salt and pepper
1 cup white wine (optional)

In a large pot, place 3 quarts water and if allowed, 1 cup white wine (dry). Also put in the 1 cup onions, carrots, peppercorns, celery and salt (3 teaspoons). Bring to a boil, and put salmon into it. Lower heat and simmer until the fish is firm. Remove and flake the fish. In a large frying pan, melt 2 tablespoons margarine and saute the mushrooms. Remove to a bowl and mix with lemon juice, a bit of the salt, and a bit of pepper. Saute the rest of the onions in 4 tablespoons margarine until clear. Add the rest of the salt and combine with the mushrooms. Heat the rest of the margarine and stir in the rice, coating thoroughly. Add the last bit of onion and the stock and bring to a boil. Cover and simmer until the rice is done. Add the dill. Stir this and the mushroom mixture into the salmon, and stir in the chopped tofu or egg. Roll out pastry on a baking tray and place this mixture on it, leaving 1 inch all around. Cover with a second layer of pastry and seal. Bake at 350°F until browned.

SALMON AND POTATO FRITTERS

2 7-ounce cans salmon
3/4 cup mashed potatoes
3 tablespoons grated onion
1 tablespoon lemon juice
1 tablespoons chopped parsley
1 teaspoon salt
1/2 teaspoon freshly ground pepper
1 egg, beaten
3/4 cup fresh bread crumbs
Oil for frying

Drain and mince salmon. Combine with remaining ingredients. Chill. Remove from refrigerator. Place mixture on floured board. Pat flat. Form into 2-inch fritters. Pour enough oil in fryer to cover fritters. Heat to 375°F. Deep fry fritters until golden brown. Drain well and serve. *Note:* Fritters can be frozen until ready to deep fry.

SHRIMP, CABBAGE AND RICE STICKS

1 pound cleaned shrimp
1/2 pound Chinese cabbage (celery cabbage)
4 tablespoons oil
1 tablespoon rice wine or dry sherry (optional)
1 1/2 teaspoons salt
1/2 teaspoon sugar
1 tablespoon soy sauce (optional)
1/2 cup chicken stock (or water)
Rice sticks

Soak the rice sticks in cold water for 5 minutes, and drain. Cut the cabbage into 1/4 inch strips. Put 2 tablespoons of the oil in a hot wok or pan, and add the shrimp. Cook for 1 minute, stirring, until they turn pink. Add the salt and wine, stir and put aside. Add the last 2 tablespoons oil, and stir fry the cabbage for 2 minutes. Add all the other ingredients, and stir until noodles are pliable. Return the shrimp to the pot and heat through. Serve.

SHRIMP HORS D'OEUVRES

1 can peeled water chestnuts
1 pound raw cleaned shrimp
1 1/2 tablespoons cornstarch
1/2 teaspoon salt
1 egg
2 tablespoons sherry

Using a blender or food processor, puree the water chestnuts, shrimp, and cornstarch (and salt). Add the egg and sherry and process until smooth. Shape into balls, and fry in oil until brown. Serve warm.

SOUPS

AVOCADO VICHYSSOISE

2 ripe avocados
1/2 pint Mocha Mix™
1 teaspoon lemon juice
Dash of onion juice
Salt and pepper to taste
5 cups chicken stock
Chopped chives

In a blender, puree avocados and add Mocha Mix, lemon juice, onion juice, and seasonings, until very smooth. Add chicken stock; chill in refrigerator. Serve very cold, with chopped chives sprinkled on top.

BARLEY SOUP

1 cup pearl barley
Cold water
2 quarts beef stock
1 tablespoon oil
1 slice onion
3 stalks celery
2 sliced carrots
2 sliced potatoes
3/4 cup fresh, diced mushrooms
1 bay leaf
Salt and pepper
Chopped dill (optional)

Soak the barley and drain. Cook in two cups stock for one and a half hours. In a big pot, cook the onions in the oil until clear, and add the rest of the stock, celery, carrots, potatoes, mushrooms and bay leaf. Cover and simmer for half and hour. Season to taste, and garnish with the dill.

BARLEY SOUP (Lamb Base)

Bones from leg of lamb, plus extra bones and meat
2 cups chopped carrots
2 cups chopped celery
1 cup chopped onions
2 quarts of water (approximately)
1 leek, sliced
1 bay leaf
1 clove of garlic, chopped
1/2 cup barley
1 1/2 teaspoon salt
2 cups strong lamb stock

Brown the meat, bones and vegetables in a shallow pan. Discard the fat and add the ingredients to a soup kettle, along with the browned bits from the pan. Add water, bring to a boil and skim. Add the rest of the ingredients and simmer for 2 hours, until the barley is tender. Add more liquid if necessary. Add seasoning, remove fat and serve.

BARLEY BEAN SOUP

1 1/2 cups lima beans
2 pounds flank steak
2 quarts water
1/4 cup pearl barley
1 onion, diced
2 teaspoons salt
2 tablespoons parsley

Rinse the lima beans and remove any debris. Cover the meat with the water and cook for 45 minutes. Add the barley, onions and beans, and simmer for 1 1/2 hours more. Add the salt and parsley, and cook for 10 minutes.

BEEF STOCK

1 1/2 pounds lean beef
2 pounds beef soupbones
2 pounds veal knuckle
3 onions, each studded with 3 cloves

12 cups water
3 carrots
3 leeks
5 stalks celery
5 sprigs parsley
7 peppercorns
2 teaspoons salt

Peel and slice the vegetables (except the parsley). Place the meat and bones in a large, heavy pot, and add the water. Bring to a boil, and skim. Add the vegetables and spices, and simmer for 3 to 3 1/2 hours. Strain through cheesecloth placed in a colander, and discard the vegetables. Put meat aside, to serve another time and refrigerate the soup. When the fat has hardened on the top, remove with a large flat spoon, so only the clear broth remains.

If you wish the soup to be really clear, you can add beaten egg whites and crushed eggshells to the soup, and boil, stirring, for 10 minutes. Allow to stand, and strain through a double-folded cheesecloth.

Or: Reheat, and allow to stand so that the particles settle on the bottom. Pour carefully through a jelly bag, leaving the sediment in the pot. This soup may be garnished with a variety of cooked diced vegetables, to make it more elegant.

BORSCHT (BEET)

2 quarts water
4 medium beets (red)
1/2 cup sugar
1/4 cup lemon juice (or more, to taste)
Salt
Boiled potatoes or sour cream

Slice the beets, and cook in the water for about an hour, until tender. Allow to cool. Add the rest of the ingredients and garnish. Serve cold (the boiled potatoes should be warm).

CHICKEN SOUP

4 to 5 pounds soup chicken or "stewing hen"
1 large onion, diced
3 carrots

3 stalks celery
2 sprigs parsley
1 tablespoon salt
Pepper to taste
Extra chicken feet or necks and backs

Cover the chicken with water. When it boils, remove scum and add vegetables. Simmer until tender, about 2 1/2 to 3 hours. Serve chicken and vegetables in soup, or strain and use chicken in other dishes.

CHINESE CHICKEN SOUP

1 soup chicken
12 cups water
3 slices ginger root
1 1/2 tablespoons salt

Place all ingredients in a large pot, Bring to a boil and skim. Reduce heat and simmer for 3 hours. Remove the fat and serve.

CHICKEN STOCK

(Alternate For Use in Chinese Cooking)

5 pounds stewing chicken (with backs and necks)
2 slices fresh ginger root, size of a quarter, peeled
1 scallion, washed and cut into pieces

Place chicken in cold water and add vegetables. Bring to a boil, skim, cover the pot and let it simmer until the chicken is very tender (2 hours). Remove the chicken, and strain soup. Remove fat.

CREAM OF CHICKEN SOUP

1 tablespoon margarine
1/4 cup flour (I use rice flour)
3 cups chicken broth
1 cup shredded cooked chicken
1 cup Mocha Mix™
Salt to taste

In a heavy saucepan, melt the margarine. Blend in the flour. Slowly add the broth and Mocha Mix™, stirring constantly with a whisk until thickened. Add the chicken and salt. Serve. This may be topped with chopped chives or parsley.

CONSOMME WITH SHERRY

Reduce 4 quarts of consomme to 2, and add 1/2 cup of sherry, just before serving.

COLD CUCUMBER SOUP

2 cucumbers
1/4 cup chopped onion
1 tablespoon chopped parsley
1/2 teaspoon salt
1/8 teaspoon freshly ground pepper
4 cups chicken broth
1 cup sour cream (dairy or non-dairy)
Chopped chives

Peel, seed and dice cucumbers. Cook cucumbers, onion, parsley, salt and pepper in chicken broth until cucumber is soft. Cool. Puree in blender or press through food mill. Blend in sour cream. Chill thoroughly. Serve in soup bowls. Garnish with chives.

FISH STOCK I

3 pounds back, head or tails of white fleshed fish
    (sea bass, striped bass, etc.)
2 cups onions, sliced
1 bay leaf
6 peppercorns
3 sprigs parsley
Pinch ground pepper
1 teaspoon salt
1 pound fillets
1 lime
Parsley for garnish

In a large soup pot, put 2 quarts of water, onions, peppercorns, bay leaf, 3 sprigs parsley, and soup fish. Bring to a boil quickly and reduce to simmer. Simmer for half an hour. If egg cannot be used to clear the soup, pour through a jelly bag into a large bowl or pot. Allow to sit so that any sediment will sink to the bottom and pour off the clear soup. Return the clear stock to a clean pot and bring to a boil. Add the fillets, and simmer until the fish is done (4 minutes). Into individual bowls, put the fish, soup, lime slices, and parsley.

FISH STOCK II

6 pounds fish, including head, bones and meat
    of a white fleshed fish
2 medium onions
2 leeks
1 bay leaf
2 teaspoons fennel
1 clove
1 teaspoon salt
12 cups water
1 cup dry white wine (optional)

Put all the ingredients into a large heavy pot. Bring to a boil, and lower the heat. Simmer for 45 minutes. Strain through cheesecloth.

FLANKEN SOUP (Beef)

3 pounds plate flank
3 carrots, sliced
3 beef bones
3 quarts water
1 onion
2 1/2 teaspoon salt
2 stalks celery, sliced
1 bay leaf

Combine the beef, bones, and water and bring to a boil. Skim, and add the rest of the ingredients. Simmer for 2 to 2 1/2 hours, until beef is tender. Strain the soup, and serve the meat with horseradish.

HAM AND BEAN SOUP

1 ham bone (with meat)
1 pound small white beans
2 quarts water
1 cup chopped celery
1 onion, chopped
2 tablespoons parsley
1 teaspoon salt
1 bay leaf

In a soup pot, bring water and beans to a boil, and cook for 2 minutes. Allow it to sit for one hour. Add the other ingredients, bring to a boil, and simmer until the beans are soft (several hours). Remove the leaf and the bone. Chop the meat into small pieces. Return the meat to the soup, and serve.

MUSHROOM-POTATO SOUP

1 1/2 pounds mushrooms, sliced
2 large onions, choppedp
6 tablespoons margarine
6 cups chicken stock
2 large scallions, chopped
3 medium potatoes, sliced and peeled
1 teaspoon salt
2 tablespoons fresh parsley, chopped
1 cup sour cream, dairy or non-dairy (optional)

In a heavy 5 quart casserole, melt 4 tablespoons margarine. In this, saute the mushrooms and onions until they are covered with the margarine. Reduce heat, and simmer for 20 minutes. Add the stock, potatoes and salt. Bring to a boil, and then simmer for 20 minutes or until the potato slices are tender. In a small heavy skillet, melt the 2 tablespoons margarine and saute the celery, scallions and parsley stirring until the celery is tender. To this mixture, add the sour cream. Use low heat. Add the contents of the pan to the soup, and serve.

SOY CREAM SOUPS

Vegetables (about 1 1/2 pounds)
Soya white sauce (Recipe in Meat Sauces section.)
Water or stock (2 to 3 cups)

Clean and trim the vegetables. Place in boiling water or stock and simmer until tender. Puree the cooked vegetables and 2 cups of the stock in a blender. In another pan, saute a small amount of onion or leek, if permitted. Puree this also. Make white sauce according to directions, add the puree, stirring constantly, and heat through. Serve.

SPLIT PEA SOUP I (Beef or Ham)

1 pound yellow split peas
1 pound green split peas
4 to 6 beef bones or hambone with meat on them
1 onion, diced
3 stalks celery, sliced
3 carrots, sliced
2 1/2 teaspoons salt

Brown the meat in the soup pot. Wash the peas, and remove any debris. Slice onion, carrots and celery. Combine all ingredients in a large soup pot and bring to a boil. Lower heat to a simmer, and cook for 2 1/2 to 3 hours (when the meat is really tender). Cut the meat from the bones and serve in the soup.

SPLIT PEA SOUP II (Chicken Base)

1 cup green split peas
2 carrots
1 cup yellow split peas
1 onion, diced (small onion)
2 pounds chicken backs and necks
2 stalks celery
1 1/2 teaspoons salt
6 cups water

Brown the meat. Wash the peas and remove any debris. Combine all ingredients in a soup pot and bring to a boil. Lower heat

108

to simmer and cook for 2 1/2 to 3 hours. Cut meat from the bones and serve in the soup.

PLAIN POTATO SOUP

6 medium potatoes
1 medium onion, finely chopped
2 tablespoons rice or barley
2 quarts water
Salt and pepper to taste
Margarine (optional)
Chopped parsley (optional)

Boil the rice (or barley) in the water. When it begins to boil, add the finely chopped onion. Cook for about an hour. Meanwhile, peel and cook the potatoes, mash them, add to the liquid mixture and season. A bit of margarine or cream (or soy cream) can be used to make the soup richer. If allowed, garnish with parsley, chopped.

POTATO SOUP

4 large potatoes
6 tablespoons shortening
1 cup celery, chopped
1 cup onions, diced
1 cup carrots, diced
2 tablespoons acceptable flour (not potato)
1 quart chicken stock
1/4 teaspoon marjoram
1/2 teaspoon salt
1/2 cup sliced mushrooms

Cook the potatoes in boiling water to cover. Peel and dice. In a large soup pot, melt the shortening and add the potatoes, onions and carrots. Cook until vegetables are lightly browned. Stir the flour into the vegetable mixture, coating well. Add the stock, spices and mushrooms, and bring the soup to a boil on high heat. Partially cover the pot and simmer for half an hour until the potatoes are done.

ZUCCHINI SOUP

3 medium or 6 small zucchini, sliced
1 onion, diced
2 cups water
2 carrots, sliced
2 potatoes or 2 tablespoons raw rice
Salt and pepper to taste
Shortening

If using potatoes, peel and dice. Saute the onions in a small amount of shortening. Add the carrots and continue cooking for 2 minutes. Add the rest of the vegetables and stir to coat. Add the water and cook until tender. If using rice, puree in a blender, adding more water if it is too thick. Add salt and pepper if allowed. Serve hot or cold.

SIZZLING RICE SOUP

Rice crusts, broken into pieces.
6 cups chicken stock
1 slice of ginger root, size of a quarter
1 cup sliced mushrooms
1/2 cup sliced water chestnuts
1/2 cup bamboo shoots, sliced
1/2 pound Napa cabbage
1/2 pound chicken meat, sliced (julienne)
3/4 cup bean curd, diced
1/2 teaspoon sesame oil
Salt to taste
Oil for frying

Bring the ginger root, stock and mushrooms to a boil and simmer for 15 minutes. Discard the ginger and all other vegetables. Bring to a boil and add the water chestnuts, bamboo shoots, cabbage, chicken, bean curd, sesame oil, and salt. Before serving, deep fry the rice crusts until they have a golden color. Add these to the soup at the table and they will sizzle and put on quite a show.

SOY BROTH FOR COOKING

1 cup soybean sprouts
5 cups water
Salt to taste

Bring the sprouts and water to a boil, and simmer for 1 hour. Add salt to taste. This makes a good base broth for Chinese cooking or for vegetarian soups.

SPINACH SOUP

8 cups chicken stock
2 pounds fresh spinach, washed and chopped
4 tablespoons margarine
1/2 teaspoon garlic, chopped
1 cup onions, chopped
1/8 teaspoon nutmeg
1 teaspoon salt
White pepper to taste

In a large pot, bring the stock to a boil. Add the spinach and simmer partially covered, for 5 or 6 minutes. In another large pot, melt the margarine, and when the foam subsides, add the onions and garlic. Saute until the onions are translucent. Add to this the broth, spinach, and the rest of the ingredients. Simmer for 10 minutes and season to taste. Serve.

TURKEY SOUP

1 turkey carcass
8 cups water
1 onion, chopped
1 teaspoon salt
2 stalks celery
1 carrot
Combine in a bag:
1 tablespoon parsley
1/2 teaspoon marjoram
1 bay leaf

Cut the turkey carcass into pieces, and put in soup pot with water. Bring to a boil and add the vegetables, salt, and spice bag. Simmer for 3 or more hours. When done, remove the meat from the bones and return to the soup. Remove the spice bag. If desired, add noodles or rice.

VEGETABLE SOUP I (Chicken Base)

2 quarts chicken broth
1 tablespoon butter or margarine
2 leeks, sliced
3 stalks celery
3 sprigs parsley
1/4 cup green pepper
1 cup lettuce
3 potatoes
1 teaspoon salt
1 teaspoon sugar

Chop all vegetables (except lettuce). In pot, melt butter and cook leaks, celery, and parsley, but do not brown. Blanch the green pepper and lettuce and drain. Pour hot chicken broth over all vegetables and simmer for 20 minutes.

VEGETABLE SOUP II (Chicken Base)

2 quarts chicken stock
3 potatoes, chopped
1 onion, chopped
2 carrots, chopped
1 package frozen stringbeans
1 green pepper, chopped
1/2 cup olive (or other) oil
1 tablespoon parsley
1 teaspoon basil
1 teaspoon salt
1 teaspoon cumin
Chicken from stock

Saute the onion, carrots and potatoes until carrots begin to soften. Add stock and green pepper and simmer until potatoes are

112

tender. Add all other ingredients and continue simmering for 10 minutes. Serve.

VEGETABLE SOUP III (Beef Based)

1 bunch spinach, washed and chopped (optional)
2 quarts beef broth
3 medium onions, chopped
3 carrots, peeled
2 large potatoes, diced
3/4 cup olive (or other) oil
2 cloves garlic (optional)
1/2 pound string beans, cooked
1 green pepper
1/2 teaspoon salt
1 1/2 teaspoon cumin
1 teaspoon basil
3 tablespoons chopped parsley
Pepper to taste

Saute the potatoes and onions in a large, heavy pot. When the potatoes are browned add the beef and broth and the carrots. Simmer. When the potatoes are tender, add the chopped pepper, string beans, basil, garlic, spinach, salt, cumin, and parsley. Simmer for 10 minutes. Serve.

VEGETABLE STOCK

1 tablespoon margarine or oil
2 carrots
2 onions
5 celery stalks (do not remove leaves)
3 quarts of water
3 sprigs parsley
1/2 cup mushroom stems (save when cooking)
1/4 cup lettuce
2 tomatoes (or substitute skin of 2 apples)

Melt the shortening in a large soup pot. Slice the vegetables (except parsley) and stir into the shortening until they are well coated. Bake this in a 350°F oven for a half hour. Add the water and simmer on the stove for 4 hours. Strain through a double layer of cheesecloth, and cool. When the fat has risen to the top, remove. Season to taste.

INSTANT DRY VEGETABLE SOUP I

Dried carrot
Dried peas
Dried celery
Dried mushrooms
Dried parsley
Other acceptable dried vegetables
Salt to taste
Dried chicken or beef

Grind each ingredient to a powder, and combine to taste. To reconstitute, add to boiling water and allow to steep for several minutes. (As a short cut, if there is a powdered broth which you can use, replace the chicken or beef with it.)

INSTANT DRY SOUP MIX II

After you have made a thick soup, such as split pea, bean, or potato soup, place a sheet of plastic wrap on a food-dryer tray. Pour the soup on this to a thickness of 1/4 inch and dry. This can then be broken up into small pieces, or ground up to a powder, and used. Reconstitute in boiling water. (See previous recipe.)

DRIED ONION SOUP MIX

1 tablespoon powdered dried onion
3 tablespoons powdered beef broth
1/4 teaspoon celery salt
3 tablespoons toasted dried chopped onions

Mix all the ingredients well. When this recipe is divided in two parts, it can be sealed in packages and used as a substitute for commercial dried onion soup mix.

MATZOH BALLS (Contains Wheat)

2 egg yolks
1/2 teaspoon salt
2 egg whites, beaten
1/2 cup matzoh meal

Beat the egg whites, until stiff. In a separate bowl, beat the egg yolks and salt until thick. Mix all ingredients. Refrigerate 1 hour or more. Wet hands, and shape batter into 1/2 inch balls. Cook in boiling water for 20 minutes, and serve in soup.

SALADS

HOT WEATHER SALAD (Grace Kim)

2 cucumbers
2 cups small shrimp and crabmeat (or 2 cups chicken, shredded)
1/2 teaspoon sugar
1 sliced carrot
A bit of water
1 tablespoon vinegar
Salt
1 teaspoon powdered mustard

Place the cucumbers, carrots, and meat on a plate, and mix the other ingredients to make a dressing. Pour the dressing over salad and serve.

CRABMEAT SALAD

3/4 pound crabmeat
2 Chinese cucumbers
2 tablespoons white vinegar
2 tablespoons soy sauce (or salt to taste)
1 teaspoon sugar
Pinch of white pepper
1 tablespoon sesame oil

Peel, seed, and shred the cucumbers. Combine all ingredients, and chill for 1/2 hour before serving.

ASPARAGUS SALAD

2 pounds fresh, thin-stemmed asparagus
4 teaspoons soy sauce
1 teaspoon sugar
2 teaspoons sesame oil

Break off the tough ends of the asparagus and slice diagonally. Wash. Drop the pieces into rapidly boiling water and cook for 1 minute. Place in ice water and then pat dry.

Combine the other ingredients. Coat asparagus with the dressing and chill before serving.

STRING BEAN SALAD

2 pounds fresh string beans, steamed and cooled
1/2 cup olive oil (or other allowed oil)
1 tablespoon tarragon vinegar (or other herb)
About a half bunch of watercress
1 tablespoon chopped dill
1 tablespoon chopped chives
Salt, pepper and sugar to taste

Mix the dressing and allow to sit while the beans cool. Mix all ingredients well and refrigerate until serving time.

COLE SLAW I

1 head of cabbage, sliced finely
2 cups cream or soy cream
1 tablespoon cider vinegar or lemon juice
1/4 cup sugar

Mix all ingredients well, chill and serve.

COLE SLAW II

1 large head of cabbage, sliced
2 medium onions, sliced
1/4 cup sugar
1/4 cup acceptable honey (light one is better)
1 tablespoon salt
1 tablespoon dry mustard
2/3 cup oil
1 cup cider vinegar
1 teaspoon celery seed

Put the cabbage and onions (sliced) in a large bowl. Mix the sugar and honey, and pour over vegetables. In a saucepan, mix the rest of the ingredients, and bring to a boil. Pour over the vegetables and mix well. Allow to sit for several hours before serving.

117

CUCUMBERS VINAIGRETTE

4 medium cucumbers, peeled and sliced
1 small yellow onion, sliced
1 tablespoon salt
2/3 cup cider vinegar
1 1/2 teaspoons sugar
3 tablespoons cold water

Spread cucumbers in a shallow pan and salt. Allow to sit for 13 to 20 minutes and drain. Toss the cucumbers with the onion slices. Mix the other ingredients and pour over the vegetables. Chill for at least an hour.

CUCUMBER ROLLS

Large cucumbers
4 cups of water
1 tablespoon salt
Stuffing (this can be a chicken-mayonnaise mixture,
    crabmeat mixture, etc).

Peel the cucumbers. Cut off the ends and cut in half across the middle. Soak in water/salt mixture for 25 minutes and drain. With a sharp knife, cut 1/8 inch spiral to the center and lay flat. Spread with the stuffing and roll up. Refrigerate for an hour, and then slice.

SWEET AND SOUR CUCUMBER SALAD

3 medium size cucumbers
1 cup water
1/2 cup vinegar
1/2 cup sugar
1 teaspoon dill seed

Cut cucumbers in half lengthwise. Scoop out seeds. Slice thin, crosswise. Place in bowl. Mix water, vinegar, sugar and dill seed and bring to a boil. Pour over cucumbers. Chill at least 2 hours. Drain and serve.

CHOPPED EGGPLANT

1 eggplant
1 dozen olives, ripe
1 onion, quartered
1/4 cup olive oil
3 tablespoons lemon juice
1/4 teaspoon sugar
Salt and pepper to taste

Bake the whole eggplant in a 350°F oven for an hour. Remove and put in cold water. When it is cool enough to handle, remove the skin. Cut into small pieces. Combine with the onion and olives, and the rest of the ingredients. Mix well and chop until all ingredients are in small pieces. Serve on lettuce leaves, chilled.

SPINACH SALAD

1 pound fresh spinach
1 teaspoon salt
2 cups water
2 1/2 tablespoons sesame seeds
2 tablespoons Shoyu (Japanese soy sauce)
1 tablespoon oil
1/2 teaspoon sugar

Wash spinach well and blanch in boiling water, covered, for about 1 minute. Drain. Cool by running cold water over spinach and drain again. Remove stems and dry leaves well with paper towels. Cut spinach leaves into small pieces. Place in salad bowl. Lightly brown sesame seeds in a frying pan. Cool. Pound them or run them through a blender. Add pulverized seeds to shoyu, sugar and oil. Mix well. Pour sauce over spinach. Toss until blended.

STUFFED PEPPER SALAD

1 medium eggplant
1/2 cup vegetable oil
1 medium, chopped onion
4 large green peppers
3/4 cup humous
Salt and pepper to taste

119

Peel, dice, and salt the eggplant. Allow to stand for 25 minutes and drain. Heat the oil and fry the eggplant. Remove the eggplant and lightly cook the onion in the oil. Allow these ingredients to cool.

Cut the top half off the peppers, and leaving the bottom half, remove the seeds and stem from the top half, and shred. Mix this with the eggplant, onion and humous. Season. Fill the pepper and shells and serve cold.

APRICOT JELLED SALAD

1 3-ounce package lemon gelatin (or equivalent made of
    agar-agar)
1/2 cup cold apricot nectar
1 cup hot apricot nectar
1 cup chopped apricots
1/2 cup peeled chopped apple or banana
1/2 cup cold water (or ice to set faster)

Dissolve the gelatin in the boiling apricot nectar. Add the cold liquid ingredients, and refrigerate until partially set. Gently mix in the fruit and refrigerate again until the mixture is set.

SALAD DRESSINGS

LEMON JUICE SALAD DRESSING

1 tablespoon olive oil
1 tablespoon lemon juice

Mix all ingredients thoroughly, and mix into green salad. This recipe may be modified by the addition of herbs, to taste (i.e. tarragon, basil, thyme).

MAYONNAISE

3 teaspoons dry mustard
3 egg yolks or egg substitute
White pepper to taste
1 1/2 cups oil

2 tablespoons tarragon (or other) vinegar
2 tablespoons lemon juice
1/2 cup chopped celery

Make mayonnaise from the ingredients indicated (or use commercial mayonnaise substitute).

EGG-FREE MAYONNAISE

1 teaspoon Ener-G™ Egg Replacer (packed)
1 tablespoon water
1 cup vegetable oil
1 teaspoon sugar
1 teaspoon salt
1 1/2 teaspoons dry mustard

Combine Ener-G™ Egg Replacer and water. Beat until peaks are formed. Add other ingredients, very slowly, one at a time, beating continuously. Makes about 1 1/2 cups egg-free mayonnaise.

EGGLESS MAYONNAISE

1/2 teaspoon salt
1/2 teaspoon dry mustard
1/2 teaspoon paprika
1 teaspoon sugar
Pinch of cayenne pepper
1 tablespoon Mocha Mix™
1 cup salad oil
1 tablespoon vinegar or 1 tablespoon each vinegar and lemon
    juice

Mix the dry ingredients. Blend in Mocha Mix™, a small amount at a time, beating after each addition. Beat in vinegar.

MOCHA MIX™ CREAM DRESSING

1 cup Mocha Mix™
3 tablespoons cider vinegar
1/2 teaspoon salt
1 teaspoon seasoned salt
1/2 teaspoon garlic salt

Combine all ingredients.
Variation:
Roquefort dressing (TRUE roquefort is made from sheep's milk). To the basic dressing add 1 tablespoon crumbled roquefort cheese.

SOYA MAYONNAISE

1/2 cup soya powder
1/2 cup water
1/2 teaspoon salt
1/2 teaspoon mustard powder
1/4 cup lemon juice (or cider vinegar)
1 cup oil

Place all ingredients except 3/4 cup of the oil in a blender and process on whip until mixed. Put blender on low speed and add the rest of the oil, a bit at a time, until it reaches mayonnaise consistency.

BREADS AND CEREALS

Recipes with EMM after the title were given by El Molino Mills.

BROWN RICE CEREAL I

1 cup brown rice, cooked as per package directions
2 teaspoons honey
1 tablespoon margarine
1/4 cup raisins
1 cup any acceptable milk or formula

Combine all ingredients in a heavy saucepan. Cook over medium heat until heated through and serve as a breakfast cereal.

BROWN RICE CEREAL II

2 cups brown rice
Salt
Water

Wash and drain rice. Put in a dry frying pan and cook at low heat until it is dry. Grind in a grain mill or processor (steel blade) until fairly fine. Cook 3 tablespoons of the ground rice in one cup of boiling water with a pinch of salt added. *For Cream of Rye Cereal:* Substitute rye berries for the rice.

FRUIT PANCAKES

Add 1/2 cup of any of these chopped fruits to pancake batter to vary a standard breakfast: dates, blueberries, dried cherries, or apple.

BARLEY GRIDDLE CAKES* EMM

1 cup barley flour
2 teaspoons baking powder
1/4 teaspoon salt
1 egg, beaten
1 teaspoon oil
1 cup cold water

Combine ingredients with 1 cup cold water. Mix thoroughly, adding more water if necessary. Bake on hot griddle.

CHESTNUT-RICE FLOUR PANCAKES

1 cup glutinous rice flour
1/4 cup water
1/4 cup brown sugar
8 ounces chestnut spread
Oil

Dissolve the sugar in the boiling water and add flour, stirring to make a dough. Roll out and cut into rounds. Fry in an oiled pan until one side is browned. Turn and brown second side. Remove to a plate, fill with spread, fold, and serve. Almost any filling may be used with these pancakes for variety.

WHOLE RYE FLOUR WAFFLES* EMM
(Wheat-Free)

3 eggs (separated)
1 1/2 cups milk
1/2 teaspoon salt
1 tablespoon dark brown sugar or honey
2 tablespoons melted butter
1 1/2 cups whole rye flour

Beat egg yolks well, add ingredients in order given. Beat egg whites until stiff but not dry and fold into batter. Bake in hot waffle iron. May also be used as pancakes. *Remarks:* 1 egg is equal in leavening power to 1/2 teaspoon baking powder.

BROWN RICE FLOUR WAFFLES* EMM
(Wheat Free)

2 cups brown rice flour
3 teaspoons baking powder
1 tablespoon brown sugar
1/2 cup chopped walnuts (optional)
2 eggs
1 1/2 cups milk
6 tablespoons oil

Beat eggs and milk together. Combine dry ingredients and add to egg and milk. Add oil. Cook in waffle iron.

SOURDOUGH PANCAKES

1 cup Jolly Joan™ Potato Mix
1 beaten egg or egg substitute
1 cup buttermilk
1 tablespoon vegetable oil
1 tablespoon brown sugar (packed)
1/2 cup instant potato flakes

Beat egg and slowly add buttermilk, then oil and brown sugar. Beat in instant potato flakes until dissolved, then beat in potato mix. Makes 12 medium size pancakes.

RICE WAFFLES

2 cups rice flour
1 tablespoon sugar
2 cups water
4 teaspoons baking powder
3 tablespoons oil or melted shortening

Sift the dry ingredients, and then add the liquid, stirring until smooth. Bake in a well-greased waffle iron, and allow to sit for a few minutes before trying to remove (otherwise it will crumble).

RICE MIX PANCAKES AND WAFFLES

1 cup Jolly Joan™ Rice Mix
1 cup milk or soy milk or soy cream
1 teaspoon egg substitute
1 tablespoon oil

Sift the dry ingredients, and then add the liquid, stirring until smooth. Bake in a well-greased waffle iron, and allow to sit a few minutes before removing (or else it may crumble).

OAT MIX PANCAKES

1 cup Jolly Joan™ Oat Mix
1 beaten egg or egg substitute
1 cup milk or soy milk
2 tablespoons melted shortening

Combine milk, beaten egg, and shortening. Add oat mix. Stir until batter is smooth. Batter should be thin. Bake on medium hot griddle. If batter thickens add milk or water. Makes 12 pancakes.

SOY WAFFLES

2 cups soy flour
3 teaspoons baking powder
2 tablespoons sugar
1/2 teaspoon salt
2 eggs, separated
5 tablespoons liquid shortening
2 cups milk or soy milk

Sift the dry ingredients thoroughly. Beat the egg yolks and add the milk. Add to the dry ingredients and mix to blend. Add the shortening. Beat the egg whites until stiff. Fold into the rest of the ingredients and bake in a waffle iron.

POTATO AND RICE MIX PANCAKES

1/2 cup Jolly Joan™ Potato
1/2 cup Jolly Joan™ Rice Mix
1 beaten egg or Jolly Joan™ Egg Replacer
1 cup buttermilk
1 tablespoon vegetable oil
1 tablespoon brown sugar (packed)

Beat egg. Add buttermilk slowly, then oil and brown sugar. Beat in potato and rice mix. Makes 12 medium size pancakes.

RICE POLISH BUTTERMILK PANCAKES

1/3 cup Jolly Joan™ Rice Polish
2/3 cup Jolly Joan™ Rice Flour
1 teaspoon baking soda
1/2 teaspoon double-acting baking powder
1/2 teaspoon salt
1 cup buttermilk
2 tablespoons oil
1 lightly beaten egg or egg substitute

Sift dry ingredients together. Add remaining ingredients and stir until blended. Drop by large spoonfuls onto lightly oiled griddle.

MATZOH BREI (Fried Matzohs)

4 matzohs
Water
4 eggs or egg substitute
1 teaspoon salt
3 tablespoon chicken fat, or margarine

Break the matzohs into pieces and soak in the water (cold) for 3 or 4 minutes. Drain well. Beat the eggs until thick and combine with matzohs and salt. Heat the shortening in a frying pan, and pour the mixture in, stirring, until bottom is browned. Serve with jelly, syrup or cinnamon sugar. *For Rice Cracker Matzoh Brei:* substitute rice crackers for the matzohs.

BAKING POWDER BISCUITS

2 cups flour (this recipe works best with wheat flour,
    although the flour mix may be used)
1 teaspoon baking powder (Cellu is corn-free)
1 teaspoon salt
1/2 tablespoon shortening
1/4 cup milk, sour cream, or water

Sift the dry ingredients into a medium bowl. Blend in the shortening. Make a well in the center and add all the liquid. Mix lightly. Place on a floured board and knead for a few seconds. Roll out a 1/2 inch thick and cut into rounds. Bake in a 450°F oven for 10 minutes. If using a soy-rice-potato starch mixture, bake at 400°F and watch carefully.

BUCKWHEAT BREAD

4 1/2 cups buckwheat flour
2 teaspoons salt
3 teaspoons baking soda
1 teaspoon baking powder
1 teaspoon dried apricots
1 cup dried prunes, pitted and soaked
1 cup raisins

127

3 cups buttermilk
1 cup brown sugar

Combine the dry ingredients in a large bowl. Coarsely chop the dried fruit and add. Mix in the buttermilk and sugar. Grease 2 loaf pans, and place equal amounts of batter in each. Bake for 1 hour in a preheated 325°F oven. Cool on a rack.

BREAD I

3 cups rice flour
1 cup potato flour
1 cup potato starch
3 cups water
2 tablespoons yeast
1 teaspoon salt
1/4 cup oil (sunflower)

Dissolve the yeast in 1/4 cup warm water. A pinch of sugar will hurry the activation, but is not necessary. Mix all ingredients thoroughly and cover with a damp cloth. Place in a warm spot to rise until trebled in bulk. Beat for 5 minutes (or 2 minutes with a heavy-duty mixer). Grease the loaf pans (each batch makes 2 loaves) and allow batter to rise in the pans, covered with a damp cloth, until doubled. Bake at 325°F until done (about 2 hours).

BREAD II

3 cups rice flour
1 cup lima bean flour
1 cup potato starch
2 1/2 cups water
2 tablespoons yeast
1/2 tablespoon salt
1/4 cup oil

Method: See directions for Bread I.

BREAD III

1 1/2 cups potato starch
1 1/2 cups potato flour

1 cup lima bean flour
2 tablespoons yeast
1 teaspoon salt
3 1/2 cups water
1/4 cup oil

Method: See directions for Bread I. (This bread does not come out as high as the rice-based breads.)

BREAD SPONGE, 72 HOUR PROCESS

Sponge:
2 potatoes
2 tablespoons brown sugar
2 teaspoons salt
1 tablespoon active dry yeast
1 cup whole wheat flour

Cook potatoes in 1 pint water and let cool. Mash and add sugar and salt. Dissolve yeast in 1/4 cup lukewarm water and let stand 15 minutes without stirring. Stir in 1 cup whole wheat flour and place in 1 quart jar (cover, but not completely). Set aside 72 hours at room temperature. Stir down each time the mixture reaches the top of the jar; repeat until it stops rising. After 72 hours, keep in ice box until ready to use.

Method:
2 cups sponge
1/2 cup oil
1/2 cup brown sugar
1 pint warm water
6 1/2 cups whole wheat flour

Combine ingredients, knead, varying amount of flour as needed, place in oiled bowl to rise. Lightly work down, place in pans, let rise a little and bake at about 350°F until done (about 50 to 60 minutes, depending on the size of the loaves).

QUICK OAT BREAD

1 20-ounce box of Ener-G™ Oat Mix
1 cup sugar

1/4 cup oil
3 cups milk/soy milk

Place sugar in large bowl. Add oil. Beat until well blended and crumbly. Add milk and oat mix. Beat until smooth, 3 to 5 minutes. Pour batter into 2 pans, approximately 8" x 4" x 2". Bake in preheated oven at 350°F for 60 to 75 minutes.

SOYA-RICE FLOUR BANANA BREAD* EMM (Wheat-Free)

1 cup brown sugar
1/4 cup oil
2 eggs (well beaten)
3 tablespoons milk
1 1/2 cup white rice flour
1/2 cup soya flour
1 teaspoon soda
3 ripe, mashed bananas
1 teaspoon salt

*Method:*Combine all ingredients. Put in warm place 1/2 hour before baking. Place in bread pans and bake at 400°F for 1 hour.

BROWN RICE FLOUR BREAD* EMM I (Yeast)

6 cups Brown Rice Flour
1/2 cup wheat germ (optional)
2 teaspoons salt
4 tablespoons brown sugar
4 tablespoons oil
1 1/2 or 2 tablespoons active dry yeast
3 cups warm water

Thoroughly mix dry ingredients. Dissolve yeast in 3 cups warm water and add oil and dry ingredients. Mix well, add more warm water to make soft mixture. Fill greased muffin tins or bread pans 3/4 full. Let stand 45 minutes. Bake in pre-heated, 350°F oven 30 minutes, until bread is brown crusted and cracks on top.

BROWN RICE FLOUR BREAD* II EMM

(With Baking Powder)

2 cups brown rice flour
1 teaspoon baking powder
1/2 teaspoon salt
2 tablespoons oil
1 tablespoon wheat germ (optional)

Combine all dry ingredients and sift. Blend in oil and make into a thin batter with about 1 cup water. Pour into a shallow greased pan and bake in a pre-heated oven at 400°F for 1 hour.

SHAKER RICE CORN BREAD

1 cup cooked rice, rubbed through a strainer
  (or put in a blender until smooth)
2 eggs (or egg substitute)
2 tablespoons shortening
1 cup white corn meal
1 cup milk (or soy milk)
1/2 teaspoon salt
1 teaspoon sugar

Add eggs and shortening to rice and beat. Add corn meal, milk, sugar, and salt and mix thoroughly. Bake in a 9 inch pan for 20 minutes at 350°F (if using soy shortening, at 325°F for a bit longer, test with a knife). Cool and serve.

ACORN BREAD

4 2/3 cups acorn flour *
2 tablespoons dry yeast
1/3 cup warm water
1/3 cup honey
2 teaspoons salt
2 tablespoons salad oil

Mix yeast with warm water to activate. When bubbling, add honey, salt and oil. Mix in flour and allow to rise, covered, in a warm place. Form loaves and bake at 350°F for 1 hour or until done. (A knife comes out clean.)

*Acorn flour: Boil the acorns for 2 to 3 hours. As the water turns brownish (and it will do this several times), change to fresh water. This removes the bitter taste. Roast the acorns, now brown in color, for 1 hour at 350°F. Grind into flour in a grain mill or processor (steel blade).

RYE BREAD* EMM (Wheat-Free)

2 cups milk
1 tablespoon oil
2 teaspoons salt
1 tablespoon active dry yeast
4 1/2 cups rye flour

Heat milk to simmering, pour over oil in bowl and add salt. When lukewarm, dissolve yeast in mixture and re-sift dough. Stir for about 5 minutes, cover with towel and let rise for about 2 hours in a warm place. Punch down and turn onto a board lightly dusted with flour. Knead 10 minutes until dough becomes springy. Shape into loaves, cover with towel and let rise until it begins to lift towel. Place in a pre-heated oven and bake at 300°F for 1 1/2 hours with a pan of hot water placed on shelf directly beneath pans of bread.

MRS. CHUANG'S STEAMED RICE YEAST BREAD

2 cups rice flour
1/4 teaspoons yeast
1 cup water
Sugar to taste

Place yeast in 2 tablespoons water with a pinch of sugar to start it bubbling. Mix the flour, water and yeast to make a batter. Add the sugar. Let the mixture sit for 3 to 4 hours in a warm place until raised (in a pilot-lit oven, or over a pan of warm water). Place in steamer and allow to sit for about 20 minutes. Then steam until done. This will take about 45 minutes to one hour, and cracks will appear on the top. Decorate with dried fruit (for example, dates). Serve warm. *Variation:* Put red bean paste or apricot jam in the middle of the risen dough for a surprise when eating.

QUICK RAISIN NUT BREAD* EMM
(Wheat-Free)

1/2 cup seedless raisins
1/2 cup walnut meats
3 teaspoons baking powder
2 cups sifted rye flour
1/2 cup milk
1/2 teaspoon salt
1/4 teaspoon cinnamon
1 egg
2 tablespoons vegetable oil
1/2 cup honey

Chop nuts coarsely and mix with raisins. Sift flour. Sift portion of flour over raisins and remainder with baking powder, salt and cinnamon. Beat egg, add honey and vegetable oil. Add dry ingredients alternately with milk, beating after each addition. Add raisins and walnut meats last. Turn into a greased loaf pan and bake at 350°F for about 1 hour. After removing from oven, let stand in pan for a few minutes, then remove to cake rack and cool.

POTATO MIX BUTTERMILK QUICK BREAD

2 cups Ener-G™ Potato Mix
2 eggs (or egg substitute)
1 cup buttermilk
2 tablespoons sugar
2 tablespoons vegetable oil

Separate eggs. Beat egg white until stiff. Set aside. Beat egg yolks, add buttermilk slowly to yolks, then sugar and oil. Beat in potato mix until smooth. Gently fold in egg whites. Pour batter into well oiled pan 8 1/2" x 4 1/2" x 2 1/2". Bake at 350°F for 40 minutes.

STICKY-RICE FLOUR DUMPLINGS

1 1/2 cups glutinous rice flour
1/2 teaspoon salt
1/2 cup boiling water (plus a bit more)

Mix dry ingredients well in a bowl. Gradually add the water, stirring constantly until it forms a stiff dough. Allow to cool, knead for 10 minutes. Roll into ropes, 1/2 inch in diameter, and cut off pieces that can be rolled in your hands to form 1/2 inch balls. Drop into boiling water, and cook. When they rise to the top, they are done. Remove and place in soup.

POTATO MUFFINS

1 1/2 cup Ener-G™ Potato Mix
1/2 cup brown sugar (packed)
1 egg (or substitute)
1/3 cup vegetable shortening
1/2 cup milk

Cream sugar and shortening together. Beat in egg, then milk. When mixture is smooth, beat in potato mix 1/2 cup at a time until smooth. Spoon into paper muffin cups 2/3 full. Bake at 375°F for 20 minutes. *Variation:* add 1/2 cup of canned blueberries.

RICE MIX MUFFINS

2 cups Ener-G™ Rice Mix
1 cup milk or soy milk
2 tablespoons honey
2 tablespoons safflower ot vegetable oil or melted shortening
1 beaten egg or egg substitute

Combine milk, egg, sugar, oil, and rice mix. Stir just enough to blend the mixture. Do not beat. Bake in muffin pans (greased on bottom only) at 425°F about 20 minutes. Makes 16 small or 8 large muffins.

EGGLESS MUFFINS

1 teaspoon Ener-G™ Egg Replacer (packed)
2 tablespoons water
2 cups sifted all-purpose flour
2 1/2 teaspoons baking powder
2 tablespoons sugar
3/4 teaspoon salt
1/4 cup oil
3/4 cup milk

Sift flour, baking powder, sugar and salt together. Combine egg replacer, milk and oil. Add all at once to flour mixture. Stir until dry ingredients are thoroughly dampened. Turn into greased muffin pans about 2/3 full. Bake at 400°F for 25 minutes or until done. Makes 10 muffins. *Variation:* 1 cup cranberries or blueberries or 1/2 cup crushed crisp bacon may be added.

RICE POLISH MUFFINS

1 cup Ener-G™ Rice Flour
1/2 cup Ener-G™ Rice Polish (sift once before measuring)
2 tablespoons granulated sugar
2 teaspoons double acting baking powder
1/2 teaspoon salt
3/4 cup of milk
1 beaten egg (or egg substitute)
1 tablespoon oil

Sift all dry ingredients together at least 3 times. Add milk, beaten egg and oil. Beat until smooth. Pour into large oiled muffin pans (8) or small oiled muffin pans (12). Fill 3/4 full. Bake at 375°F for 18 to 20 minutes.

SOYA MUFFINS* EMM (Wheat-Free)

2 eggs separated
3 tablespoons brown sugar
1 tablespoon grated orange peel
1 tablespoon melted butter or margarine
2 teaspoons baking powder
1 cup milk
1 1/2 cups soya flour
1/4 cup raisins
1/4 cup chopped walnut meats
Pinch of salt

To beaten egg yolks, add brown sugar and grated orange peel, then add melted butter. Add flour, baking powder and salt sifted together, alternately with the milk. Add stiffly beaten egg whites. Then add raisins and chopped walnut meats. Bake at 325°F for 35 minutes.

BROWN RICE FLOUR MUFFINS* EMM
(Wheat-Free)

1 cup brown rice flour (sift before measuring)
1 1/2 teaspoon baking powder
1/4 cup dark brown sugar
1/4 teaspoon salt
1 egg (beaten)
1/2 cup milk
4 tablespoons oil

Sift dry ingredients together. Beat egg, add milk and oil, blend into dry ingredients, but do not beat. Bake in well greased muffin tins for 15 minutes in a 450°F oven. This recipe makes 6 large or 12 small muffins. May also be made and shaped as a loaf of bread.

HONEY MUFFINS* EMM (Wheat-Free)

2 cups barley flour
2 teaspoons baking powder
1 teaspoon soda
1/2 teaspoon salt
1/4 cup cream or canned milk
2 tablespoons vegetable oil
2 tablespoons honey (overflowing)
1 teaspoon vanilla
2 eggs
1/2 cup dark brown sugar

Combine milk, vegetable oil, honey and vanilla in bowl. Add beaten eggs and sugar. Mix well. Sift dry ingredients and add to liquid mixture. Pour or spoon into greased muffin tins (mixture is the consistency of cookie dough). Makes one dozen. Bake at 400°F for 20 minutes. If you like a cookie with a cake texture, add coconut, nuts, raisins, or dates to the above recipe and drop onto a greased cookie sheet and bake 8 minutes at 375°F.

MILLET-BARLEY-SOYA MUFFINS* EMM
(Wheat-Free)

1/2 cup millet flour
1/2 cup barley

1/4 cup soya flour
1/2 teaspoon salt
1 egg
3 teaspoons baking powder
1/3 cup water
1 tablespoon oil
4 tablespoons honey

Sift flours before measuring. Mix dry ingredients. Beat egg and add oil, honey and water. Blend with dry ingredients, mix lightly. Bake at 375°F for 25 minutes.

BARLEY MUFFINS* EMM (Wheat-Free)

2 cups barley flour
2 teaspoons baking powder
1 teaspoon baking soda
Pinch of salt (scant)
1/2 cup dark brown sugar
2 eggs
1/4 cup cream (add water if moist batter is desired)

Sift dry ingredients together. Add combined egg and liquid, beat thoroughly. Makes 1 dozen muffins. Bake at 400°F for 25 minutes.

SOYA-RICE FLOUR COFFEE CAKE* EMM (Wheat-Free)

1/2 cup soya flour
1 1/2 cups white rice flour
4 teaspoons baking powder
1/2 teaspoon salt
4 tablespoons brown sugar
2 eggs, beaten lightly
1 cup milk
1 teaspoon cinnamon
1 tablespoon vanilla

Mix all ingredients, bake in a cake pan for 35 minutes at 350°F.

GLUTINOUS RICE-FLOUR DOUGH

1 1/2 cups boiling water
2 1/4 cups glutinous rice flour
1/4 cup potato starch flour
3/4 teaspoon salt
1/2 teaspoon sugar

Start the water boiling. Combine the other ingredients well, and pour in the boiling water. Mix, and knead for several minutes until smooth and elastic. If it gets too sticky, add a bit of potato starch flour, and be sure that the board on which you are kneading is floured.

SWEET (GLUTINOUS) RICE DOUGH

2 cups glutinous rice flour
6 tablespoons brown sugar
1/2 cup plus 2 tablespoons boiling water

Bring the water to a boil in a small pot. Pour this over the flour, stirring constantly. Knead on a floured board until smooth. *For Sweet Rice Pastries*: Roll dough out and cut in circles. Place a spoonful of sweet red bean paste in the middle and fold in half. Crimp the edges to seal tightly. Deep fry in medium oil for aproximately 3 minutes. Turn as they cook.

SCOTCH SHORTBREAD

1/2 cup sifted Ener-G™ Rice Polish
1 1/2 cups Ener-G™ Rice flour
1 cup butter or margarine
1/2 cup powdered sugar
1/4 teaspoon salt

Place all ingredients in bowl and beat until well blended. Spread layer of powdered sugar on board. Then place one-fourth of short bread mix on board. Press out into a circle 1/2 inch to 3/4 inch thick. Place in baking sheet which has been covered with aluminum foil or brown paper. With sharp knife cut into 8 wedges just half way through. Repeat this procedure for the other three parts of shortbread mix. Bake at 325°F for 30 minutes.

RICE-POTATO CRACKERS

1/4 cup potato starch flour
2 cups brown rice flour
1 teaspoon salt
1/2 cup shortening
3/4 cup water

Mix the dry ingredients, and then add the shortening and water. Mix thoroughly. Roll quite thin between sheets of foil. Place on a baking sheet and remove the top foil sheet. Bake at 320°F until light brown. *Note:* Before baking, mark for cutting with a knife.

RICE AND PEANUT CRACKERS

2 cups rice flour
1 tablespoon corn starch
1/2 medium onion, grated
1 teaspoon coriander
1 cup water
1 cup coconut milk
1 cup chopped unsalted peanuts
Salt to taste
Oil for frying

Mix all dry ingredients and nuts. Add the onions, then the liquid, stirring to make a smooth batter. Drop into hot oil and fry until light brown.

CHURROS

2 cups water
2 cups flour (wheat)
1 teaspoon salt
Oil for deep frying
Powdered sugar

Boil the water and salt over high heat. Remove from heat and add the flour, beating to form a thick paste. Cool. Heat the oil to 400°F (or highest non-smoking heat) and push the paste through a pastry press, using star shape to form 4 inch strips. Fry, turning until light brown. Remove, drain, and dust with powdered sugar.

FRIED CORN DODGER

2-3 cups boiling water
1 tablespoon bacon fat (or other frying medium)
3 cups white cornmeal
2 teaspoons salt

Mix the dry ingredients in a large bowl. Add boiling water slowing, mixing until a dough is made. Add the bacon fat and mix well. Grease a baking sheet, and heat in a 450°F oven. When it is sizzling hot, put the batter by large spoonfuls on the sheet. Pat with a spoon to even out. Bake at 450°F for 20 minutes, and reduce the heat to 350°F. Bake until golden.

SHAKER CORNMEAL WAFERS

3/4 cups boiling water
1 teaspoon salt
2/3 cup white or yellow corn meal
1 teaspoon sugar
2 tablespoons margarine
Optional: celery seeds, poppy seeds, herbs

Pour boiling water over meal, sugar and margarine. Mix well. Drop onto greased baking sheet (mixture will spread), sprinkle with seeds or herbs, and bake at 425°F until light brown (10 minutes). Allow to cool before removing from baking sheet.

TORTILLAS

2 1/3 cup masa harina (corn)
1 teaspoon salt
1 1/2 cups cold water

Combine the dry ingredients in a bowl and add the water (1 cup at first) slowly, mixing well, until you have a firm dough. Break off pieces and roll into 1 1/2 inch balls. Roll out (or use a tortilla press) to make a 6 inch tortilla on waxed paper. On a hot ungreased griddle, fry each tortilla until it is light brown.

BEVERAGES

APRICOT NECTAR

1 quart apricots
1/2 cup sugar
1 quart water
1 tablespoon lemon juice (or 2 teaspoons ascorbic acid)

Wash and pit the fruit. Boil the fruit in the water for 5 minutes. Strain. Add sugar and lemon juice (or ascorbic acid) and bring to a boil. Seal in jars to keep or cool and drink.

BEEF TEA

1 pound beef (stronger-flavor cut)
2 cups water
3/4 teaspoon salt
1 sprig parsley
2 celery leaves

Cut the meat into small pieces, and place in cold water. Add other ingredients. Cover pot tightly and simmer for 3 1/2 hours. Strain and serve.

CRANBERRY JUICE

4 cups cranberries
4 cups water
1 1/2 cups water
Sugar

Since most commercial cranberry juice contains corn syrup or honey, if you are unable to find the "lo-cal" type, you might wish to make your own. Boil the washed cranberries in 4 cups of water for 15 minutes. Let drip through a jelly bag, and then reboil the pulp in the 1 1/2 cups water. Pass this through a jelly bag also. Mix. Add 1/2 cup sugar to every 2 cups juice and bring to a boil. Put into sterile jars and seal.

CRANBERRY ICED TEA

1 quart iced tea
1 quart cranberry juice

Mix together and pour over ice cubes.

GRAPE JUICE

1 cup water
Up to 6 cups sugar, depending on grapes used
Ascorbic acid, as per instructions

Place grapes and water in large pot, and simmer until pulp rises to the top (about half an hour). Strain through a jelly bag. Add sugar, boil to dissolve, and place in sterilized jars. Add ascorbic acid according to amount of juice. Seal according to canning instructions. To use, dilute the juice by 50%.

PEAR NECTAR

1 quart pears
1/2 cup sugar
1 quart water
1 tablespoon lemon juice (or 2 teaspoons ascorbic acid powder)

See method for Apricot Nectar.

POMEGRANATE COOLER

1 large pomegranate
3 cups water
1 sliced lemon
3/4 cups sugar

Cut pomegranate in half. Remove seeds. Add seeds to water with half the lemon slices. Bring to a boil. Boil 15 minutes. Add sugar. Boil another 5 minutes. Strain. Add juice of the remaining lemon. Chill and serve in chilled glasses.

RICE TEA

1 cup rice
Water

In a skillet, toast the rice over low heat until slightly browned. Let cool, and keep in an airtight container. Use 1 tablespoon in a teapot with 4 cups of boiling water. Allow to steep for a few minutes.

DESSERTS

Recipes with EMM after the title were given by El Molino Mills.

SUGARED AGAR-AGAR

1/4 ounce agar-agar (in sticks or in flakes)
3 cups water
3/4 cup white sugar (cane or beet)
2/3 cup brown sugar
1 1/2 cups water

Bring the water and the 3/4 cup sugar to a boil, and add the agar-agar (if sticks, cut into 3/4 inch pieces). Simmer for 20 minutes, stirring intermittently. Pour the hot mixture through a strainer into a flat-bottomed pan, and allow to cool. Bring the brown sugar and water to a boil and simmer until the sugar is dissolved. Cut the cooled agar-agar into shapes, and place in dishes. Pour the syrup over it.

WATER CHESTNUT SQUARES

10 ounces water chestnut powder
6 cups sugar cane juice
2 cups water
8 ounces sugar
2 ounces lard or Crisco (solid shortening)

Put the water chestnut powder in a bowl and mix with 2 cups cane juice. Put the water in a deep saucepan. Add sugar and 4 cups of the cane juice. Bring to a boil, add the lard or Crisco and mix. Add the water chestnut mixture slowly, stirring. Pour mixture into a greased pan and steam 40 minutes over high heat. Let cool and refrigerate. Cut into serving pieces.

This is a Chinese confection, and is quite sweet. The ingredients are usually available in Oriental food stores.

PIES AND PASTRIES

FLUFFY APRICOT PIE

1/2 cup apricot nectar
1/2 cup sugar
1/4 cup cold water
1 tablespoon unflavored gelatin or agar-agar
1/4 teaspoon salt
1 1/2 tablespoons lemon juice
1 cup pureed apricots
1 container (6 ounces) heavy cream, whipped,
     or substitute whipped soy cream
1 baked pie crust

Soak the gelatin in water for 5 minutes. Combine all ingredients except cream in a saucepan and simmer until the gelatin is completely dissolved. Cool. When the mixture is partially thickened, fold into the whipped cream and put into pie shell. Chill well and serve.

BLUEBERRY PIE

3 cups blueberries, washed
1/2 cup sugar
1/8 teaspoon salt
1 tablespoon tapioca, for thickening
Pastry for 2 crusts (top and bottom)

Put bottom crust in 8 inch pie pan. Gently mix together the rest of the ingredients and pour into crust. Put top crust in place and bake at 350°F for 45 minutes. Baking at 325°F for longer time (55 minutes) may be necessary if the crust is made with soy and rice flour.

EGG-FREE CUSTARD PIE FILLING* EMM

1/3 cup Ener-G™ Egg Replacer (packed)
1/2 cup sugar
1 teaspoon vanilla
1/2 cup milk

2 1/2 cups scalded milk or soy milk
1 baked 9-inch pie shell
1/8 teaspoon salt
Nutmeg

Scald milk. In large bowl, stir egg replacer into 1/2 cup milk until smooth. Add sugar, salt and vanilla, stirring until smooth. Gradually add hot scalded milk. Pour into custard cups or baked pie shell. Sprinkle top with nutmeg. Cool.

EGG-FREE LEMON PIE FILLER* EMM

1/4 cup Ener-G™ Egg Replacer
1 cup sugar
1/4 teaspoon salt
1 1/2 cups hot water
1/3 cup lemon juice
2 tablespoons lemon rind
1 baked 9-inch pie shell

In double boiler combine egg replacer, sugar, and salt. Stir with rubber spatula until thoroughly blended. Add water, lemon juice, and lemon rind. Continue stirring until smooth and thick. When dropped from spatula, mixture should mound. Remove from heat. Stir for 5 minutes to cool. Pour into pie shell. Let cool thoroughly. Refrigerate at least 2 hours before serving.

APRICOT COBBLER

1 1/2 pounds fresh apricots, cut in half and pitted
1 cup flour mix (or acceptable flour)
1 cup sugar
1/4 cup margarine
1 teaspoon egg substitute
1/2 teaspoon salt
2 teaspoons baking powder (if not using flour mix.
    If using flour mix use 1 teaspoon baking powder).

Place the apricots in a baking dish. Mix all other ingredients until they have the consistency of cornmeal. Sprinkle over the apricots. Bake at 350°F for a half hour. Top with whipped cream or soy cream.

PEAR COBBLER

Follow the directions for Apricot Cobbler, on previous page, substituting firm ripe pears.

PEAR TARTS

6 large pears
Sugar
1/8 teaspoon cloves

Peel and wash the pears, cut in half and remove the seeds and stem. In a heavy saucepan, cook until mushy over medium heat, and puree. Measure, and use half the quantity of sugar that you have in pears. Boil the sugar with 1/4 cup water until it forms a thread when dripped from a spoon. Add the pears and continue cooking for a few minutes to blend well. Add the cloves and cool. Put into already baked pastry shells.

TOFU PIE

1 1/2 pounds tofu (soy bean curd)
1/2 cup brown sugar
2 teaspoons egg substitute (or 2 eggs)
2 tablespoons lemon juice
1 teaspoon vanilla
2 ripe bananas
8 ounces pineapple, drained
Acceptable crumb crust (see recipes)

Drain the tofu, and combine all the ingredients in a food processor or blender (except the crust). Do this in batches which are small enough for the individual machine. Pour into cooled crust, and bake at 325°F for 45 minutes or until a knife comes out clean. Cool, and refrigerate.

OAT MIX PIE CRUST

2 cups Ener-G™ Oat Mix
7 to 8 tablespoons cold water
1/2 cup shortening

Cut shortening into mix (finely). Add water. Work with hands until soft dough is formed. Cut dough into 2 parts and roll out thin on floured board. Press pastry to make fancy edge. Use fork to prick bottom to prevent buckling. Bake in preheated oven at 400°F for 23 to 25 minutes. Recipe makes enough pastry for one 9-inch, 2-crust pie or two 8-inch pie shells.

RICE FLOUR PIE CRUST* EMM

For one 9-inch pie
1 cup brown rice flour
1 tablespoon potato flour
1/2 teaspoon salt
4 tablespoons margarine
4 tablespoons ice water

Combine rice flour, potato flour and salt. Cut in margarine with pastry blender to a fine texture. Add ice water to form a soft dough. Pat dough evenly into pie pan. Bake 15 minutes or until nicely browned in 425F° oven.

CRUMB CRUST

1 1/2 cups cookie crumbs (use a recipe for a crisp cookie)
3 tablespoons margarine

Mix the crumbs, margarine and flavoring. Press on the bottom and sides of a pie pan. Bake in a 350°F oven for about 10 minutes. Cool before filling.

Variations: Add 1 teaspoon vanilla or 1 teaspoon instant coffee powder

CAROB HOT WATER PASTRY

1 cup sifted flour
1/2 teaspoon salt
3 tablespoons sugar
3 tablespoons carob powder
1/4 cup boiling water
1/3 cup shortening
1/4 teaspoon vanilla extract

Sift the flour, salt, and sugar and carob together. Add the hot water to the shortening and beat until smooth. Add the vanilla. To this mixture, add the sifted ingredients and mix. Form into a ball and roll out on a floured board. Place in a pie pan and prick all over with a fork. Bake in a 350°F oven for 10 minutes or until done. Cool before filling.

As this pastry has a cookie-like texture it can be used with a filling, in several layers, to form a torte. This can be topped with slivers of carob.

FRUITS

FROZEN APRICOT TORTE

2 cups fresh apricots, pitted and chopped
1 cup sugar
1 tablespoon lemon juice (or 1 teaspoon ascorbic acid)
1 cup whipping cream (dairy or non-dairy) whipped
1 cup coarse macaroon crumbs (or other crumb crust
    — see recipes)

Add the sugar and lemon juice to apricots. Fold in whipped cream. Place half of the crumbs in the bottom of a quart refrigerator tray. Pour in the apricot mixture and top with the remaining crumbs. Freeze until firm.

AVOCADO DESSERT

4 ripe avocados
1/2 cup lime juice
1/3 cup powdered sugar
1 lime, thinly sliced

Place the first three ingredients in a blender or processor and mix well. Chill and garnish with lime wedges and serve.

AVOCADO CREAM

3 large peeled, chopped avocados
5 tablespoons sugar

1 teaspoon vanilla
Juice and grated rind of 1 lemon
Pinch of salt

Blend all ingredients until smooth. Chill and serve.

CRANBERRY ICE

2 cups cranberries
2 1/2 cups water
3 cups sugar
1 tablespoon gelatin or agar-agar
1 tablespoon lemon juice (if allowed)

Boil the cranberries in the water, and cook until the berries are soft. Strain the mixture and then return to a pot. Add the sugar and simmer until the sugar is dissolved. Place in an ice cream freezer, and follow manufacturer's directions for freezing.

BAKED APPLES

6 green apples (or golden delicious, in which case,
    use a bit less sugar)
4 tablespoons brown sugar or maple sugar
3 tablespoons margarine
1 cup boiling water

Pare and slice the apples. Place in a baking dish. Mix the other ingredients and boil for a few minutes until well blended. Pour over the apples and bake in 350°F oven for 20 minutes or until apples are soft. Baste during baking.

SHAKER BAKED APPLES

6 green apples
1/4 teaspoon cinnamon, if allowed
1/3 cup honey
Apple cider (boiled until concentrated)
1/4 teaspoon cloves

Into a greased baking dish, put sliced green apples, and sprinkle with cinnamon and cloves. Add honey and enough cider to be 1/2 inch deep. Bake in a 350°F oven for 20 minutes.

SHAKER HONEYED APPLE RINGS

2 cups honey
1 cup vinegar
1 teaspoon cinnamon
1 teaspoon salt
2 quarts apples, cored and sliced in rings

Heat the liquid ingredients and spices in a deep skillet and cook the apple rings in the mixture, a few at a time, until they are transparent. Remove to a plate and pour any syrup in the pan over them. Use as a garnish with meat.

SHAKER APPLESAUCE*

2 pounds apples
1 cup boiled cider (make from 1 quart cider)

Peel and cut the apples in quarters. If not a juicy variety, add a little water. Add the cider and simmer until apples are done. Force through a sieve.

*This is good applesauce if the apples you are using are too tart to be used without sugar.

BAKED BANANAS

1 banana per person
Margarine
Honey to taste, or brown sugar

Peel and halve the bananas. Brush them with the margarine, or with a mixture of margarine and sweetener. Put on a baking sheet or in a shallow pan in which they will fit in 1 layer. Bake at 375°F for 15 minutes. Serve.

FRIED BANANAS

2 tablespoons margarine
1 banana per person
Optional: 1 teaspoon grated lime
1 teaspoon lime juice and 1/2 teaspoon sugar

151

Fry the bananas over low heat until tender, turning once. Use either plain margarine, or margarine plus optional ingredients.
This is usually served as an accompaniment to the entree, or as dessert.

MIXED FRUIT TZIMMES

Any combination of these:
1/2 pound dried pears
1/2 pound dried apricots
1/2 pound dried prunes
1/2 pound dried peaches

Plus:
1/2 pound dried raisins or currants
3/4 cup brown rice
3 cups water, boiling
1/2 cup honey
1/3 cup margarine
1 1/2 teaspoon grated lemon peel
3 tablespoons lemon juice
1/2 teaspoon salt
1/4 teaspoon cinnamon (optional)
2 tablespoons acceptable flour or other thickener
2 tablespoons margarine
1 cup water
Note: Ascorbic acid may be substituted for lemon peel and lemon juice.

Wash and soak the fruit for 1 hour in the boiling water (bring water to a boil, remove from heat and soak fruit). Add the rest of the ingredients, except flour, margarine and 1 cup water, to the fruit and bring to a boil. Simmer for 3/4 of an hour, or until the rice is done. In a small saucepan, heat 2 tablespoons acceptable flour (not potato) until lightly browned. Add 2 tablespoons margarine and when melted, add 1 cup water. Bring to a boil and cook for 2 minutes until smooth and thick. Add to fruit. Bring back to a boil and cook until liquid is thick. Put into a casserole and brown lightly under broiler.

PEACH BAVARIAN

1 pint sliced peaches
1 3-ounce package lemon gelatin
1 cup boiling water
1/4 teaspoon salt
2 cups whipped topping
1 tablespoon sugar

Drain the peaches, reserving 1/3 cup of the syrup. Chop the peaches. Dissolve the gelatin, sugar and salt in boling water, and stir. When dissolved, add the reserved syrup and chill until thickened. Blend the gelatin with the whipped topping, and fold in the peaches. Chill until firm (several hours) and unmold.

GELATINS

APPLE GELATIN

2 tablespoons gelatin or agar-agar
1/2 cup cold water
1 cup boiling water
1 teaspoon lemon juice (or water plus ascorbic acid)
2 cups apple cider (which has been boiled and concentrated)
Sugar to taste

Soak the gelatin in cold water, and add boiling water to dissolve. Add cider and lemon juice. Taste, and if necessary, add sugar. Cool and allow to set.

SHAKER BOILED CIDER GELATIN

2 tablespoons unflavored gelatin (or agar-agar)
1/2 cup cold water
1 cup boiling water
1 teaspoon lemon juice
2 cups boiled cider
Sugar to taste (optional)

Soak the gelatin in cold water for 5 minutes. Add the boiling water and stir to dissolve. Cool. Add the cider and lemon juice.

Chill and serve. (If you wish it to be sweeter, add the sugar when you add the boiling water.)

LEMON GELATIN DESSERT

1/2 cup unflavored gelatin or agar-agar
1 cup cold water
2 cups boiling water
Juice of 3 lemons
3/4 cup sugar

Soak the gelatin in the cold water for 5 minutes. Add the boiling water and sugar and stir until dissolved. Add the lemon juice and mix. Chill until set.

COFFEE GELATIN

2 tablespoons unflavored gelatin or agar-agar
1/2 cup cold water
4 cups hot strong coffee
1/2 cup sugar
1 teaspoon vanilla extract
Whipped cream (soy or dairy)

Soak the gelatin in cold water. Add to the hot coffee and stir to dissolve. Add the sugar, stir, then add vanilla. Pour into a prepared mold, and refrigerate. To serve, top with whipped cream.

PUDDINGS

APPLE BREAD PUDDING

6 large green apples
2 cups bread crumbs (fine)
2/3 cup margarine
1 cup sugar
1 teaspoon nutmeg, if allowed
1 cup cold water

Pare and chop apples. On a baking dish put layers of apples, crumbs, etc. On this, dot the margarine and sugar. Repeat until you have added all your ingredients, and then add your cold water. Bake 30 minutes at 350°F. Serve. The taste will change slightly depending on the bread which is used. If you cannot find green cooking apples, golden delicious may be used, but use less sugar.

RED BEAN PUDDING

1 pound red beans
8 cups water
2 cups sugar
1/2 cup lard or solid shortening
14 ounces rice flour mixed with 3 cups water

Wash and drain the beans. Pour water into a pot and add beans. Bring to a boil over medium heat and simmer for 1 hour until beans are tender. Add sugar and cook until melted. Add shortening and stir well. Sift the rice flour into a mixing bowl and mix into a batter with the 3 cups of water. Stir the batter into the bean mixture gradually until well blended. Pour into a greased cake pan and steam in a steamer over high heat for 1 hour. Slice and serve.

COCONUT CREAM PUDDING

4 cups coconut cream (See recipe on Page 21.)
3/4 cup rice flour
1 teaspoon salt
1/2 cup powdered sugar

Combine the flour, 1 cup coconut cream and salt in a bowl. Add sugar. Scald the rest of the cream, and then slowly add the mixture, stirring. Simmer, stirring until the mixture is thick. Pour into bowls or mold and refrigerate for 4 hours or more. Unmold and serve. To vary, add vanilla when cooked.

POTATO STARCH PUDDING

Apple:
2 pounds tart red apples, sliced
3 cups cold water

1/2 cup sugar
1 tablespoon potato starch in 1 tablespoon water

Apricot:
1/2 pound dried apricots
4 1/2 cups water
4 tablespoons sugar
1 tablespoon potato starch in 1 tablespoon water

Put the fruit in a large saucepan with the water. Bring to a boil and simmer the fruit for 15 minutes, or until tender. Put fruit through a sieve, and add the sugar. Return to the pan and bring to a boil. Reduce the heat to medium and add the starch mixture. Cook, stirring for 3 minutes until it comes to a boil and begins to thicken. Refrigerate for 4 hours. Serve.

RICE PUDDING

1/3 cup uncooked rice
3 cups milk or Mocha Mix™
1/3 cup granulated sugar
1/2 teaspoon salt
2/3 cups raisins
Nutmeg (optional)

Combine the first four ingredients pour into a greased baking dish. If desired, sprinkle with nutmeg. Bake in a slow oven for 2 1/2 hours, stirring occasionally during the first hour. Add the raisins and finish baking.

SHAKER SUMMER PUDDING

Shortening
4 cups berries (blueberries, blackberries)
Bread (whichever bread is acceptable)
Sugar to taste

In a greased pan, place bread with crusts cut off, in a layer. On this, add a layer of berries, sugar, and repeat until ingredients are used up. Refrigerate and allow to stand overnight. Unmold, slice and serve.

APRICOT PUDDING

1 1/2 cups dried apricots
4 cups water
1/3 cup sugar
Pinch of salt
1 tablespoon potato flour
1 tablespoon cold water

Combine the apricots and 4 cups water in a saucepan. Bring to a boil and simmer for 15 minutes or until tender. Puree in blender and return to saucepan. Add the sugar and salt. Cook the puree until it boils, and reduce heat. Mix the flour and water and add to puree. Bring to a boil and stir until it thickens. Chill for several hours.

PRUNE PUDDING

Follow the directions for Apricot Pudding. Use dried pitted prunes.

CARROT PUDDING

1 cup grated carrots
1 cup grated potatoes
1 cup sugar
1 cup flour
1 teaspoon cloves
1 teaspoon cinnamon
1 teaspoon nutmeg
1 teaspoon baking soda
1/2 teaspoon salt
1 cup chopped nuts (optional)
3 tablespoons liquid coffee
1 tablespoon oil

Mix all ingredients well. Fill a mold 3/4 full and steam for three hours. Serve with lemon sauce.
Alternate method: Bake in a greased baking dish at 300°F for 1 hour or until knife comes out clean.

COOKIES

CHEWY BROWN SUGAR COOKIES

2 cups light brown sugar
Pinch of salt
1/8 teaspoon baking soda
2 beaten eggs, or egg substitute
1 cup chopped nut meats (including soy nuts)

Thoroughly mix together all ingredients. Pour into a 9 inch cake pan and bake at 250°F for about 55 minutes. Cut into squares after they have cooled.

COOKIE DOUGH (Good for Hamentaschen)

3 cups acceptable flour or mix
3 eggs or egg substitute (or 6 ounces tofu)
1 1/2 teaspoons baking powder
1/2 cup oil
1 teaspoon vanilla
1/4 cup water
1/3 cup sugar
1/2 teaspoon salt

Combine the dry ingredients. In mixer, mix the eggs and oil, adding the sugar and vanilla gradually. Add water. Combine and mix the two mixtures. Roll out on a floured board and cut into circles. Place 1 teaspoon filling in the middle of each circle, and fold in edges to form a triangle (or any other shape desired). Bake at 350°F for 10 minutes until lightly browned.

NUT-JAM COOKIES

1 1/2 cups ground walnuts
2/3 cup sugar
2 egg whites
1 jar apricot jam

Heat the oven to 350°F. Butter and flour a baking sheet, removing the excess flour. In a mixing bowl, combine the walnuts and the sugar, Lightly beat the egg whites, and add half to this mixture, forming a paste. Roll the paste into long rolls about an inch in diameter. Make a channel in each of the rolls leaving a bit at the ends of each. Place on baking sheet and bake in the middle of the oven until browned. Heat the jam and when the rolls are removed from the oven, pour into the channels. Allow to cool, and cut into slices to serve.

PUFFED RICE COOKIES

7 cups puffed rice (brown)
1/2 cup margarine
2 cups sugar
1 teaspoon vanilla
1/3 cup soy nuts (optional)
1/4 cup raisins (optional)

Spread the puffed rice, soy nuts and raisins in a large baking pan, and put into a 200°F oven while making the syrup. Melt the margarine in a small pot over medium heat, and add the sugar and vanilla, stirring until syrup is dissolved and the syrup is dissolved and the syrup thickens (5 minutes). Pour over the warm rice and nut mixture and blend quickly. Press into pan and allow to cool. Cut into pieces.

GOLDEN RAISIN OATMEAL CRISPS

1 cup raisins
2 eggs or egg substitute
2 cups quick-cooking oatmeal
1 cup packed light brown sugar
1/2 cup salad oil
1 teaspoon salt
1 teaspoon vanilla
1 cup shredded coconut

Rinse and drain the raisins. Beat the eggs lightly. Add the remaining ingredients and blend well. Drop by spoonfuls onto greased baking sheet and flatten out with the back of a spoon into 2 1/2 inch rounds. Bake in a 350°F oven for 8 to 10 minutes or until golden brown. Cool.

159

RICE FLOUR BROWNIES

2 eggs, well beaten
1 cup sugar
1/2 cup Ener-G™ Rice Mix
2 squares chocolate melted with 1/4 pound butter or margarine
   (or equivalent amount of carob)
1 teaspoon vanilla
1 cup nuts (or soy nuts), chopped (optional)

Combine the ingredients in order given, beating well. Spread in an 8" x 11" floured pan. Bake for 30 to 35 minutes at 350°F.

POTATO MIX BROWNIES

1 cup Ener-G™ Potato Mix
1 cup sugar
2 squares chocolate (melted)
2 eggs or egg substitute
1/3 cup soft margarine
1 teaspoon vanilla
1/2 cup walnuts

Beat eggs well, beat in sugar gradually. Then beat in soft margarine and melted chocolate. Mix in potato mix until smooth. Stir in vanilla and nuts. Pour batter into oiled and dusted 8" x 8" x 2" square pan (dust with potato mix). Bake at 350°F about 35 to 40 minutes. Cool in pan, then cut.

RICE POLISH DROP COOKIES EMM

1 1/2 cups rice polish
1 1/2 cups sifted rice flour
1/2 teaspoon baking soda
1 teaspoon salt
1 teaspoon cinnamon
1/2 cup brown sugar (packed)
1 egg or egg substitute
1 teaspoon vanilla
3/4 cup milk
1 cup nuts (optional)
1/4 cup shortening

Sift rice polish once before measuring. Sift together rice polish, rice flour, soda, salt, cinnamon. In a separate bowl, cream shortening and sugar; add egg and vanilla. Beat until light and fluffy. Alternately beat in milk and flour mixture. Stir in nuts. Drop from teaspoon onto oiled baking sheet. Bake at 375°F for 15 minutes. Makes about 4 dozen.

SUGAR NUT COOKIES

2 cups light brown sugar
2 eggs, beaten
1 cup chopped nuts (or soy nuts)
1/8 teaspoon salt
1/8 teaspoon baking soda

Mix the dry ingredients. Add the eggs and mix well. Pour into a pan so the mixture is about a half inch thick. Bake at 250°F for almost an hour. Cool, and cut into squares.

PRUNE FILLING FOR COOKIES

1 pound prunes
4 tablespoons honey
2 tablespoons lemon juice (or 1/8 teaspoon ascorbic acid)

In a heavy pot, put prunes and water to cover. Bring to a boil, lower heat, and simmer 10 minutes. Cool and remove the pits. Puree prunes, and add the other ingredients. Mix well, and use in cookies and pastries.

BABY CEREAL RAISIN COOKIES

2 cups baby-food rice cereal
1/2 teaspoon salt
1/4 cup water
1 cup brown sugar
2 tablespoons margarine
1 tablespoon baking powder
1 egg, beaten lightly
1/4 cup raisins

161

Combine all the ingredients except the raisins, and beat until smooth. Add the raisins and mix. Drop by spoonfuls on an oiled baking sheet and bake at 350°F until golden (about 10 minutes).

SUGAR COOKIES

2 cups Ener-G™ Oat Mix
1/2 cup shortening
1 1/2 cups sugar
2 eggs or egg substitute
1 teaspoon vanilla
1 teaspoon caraway seed (optional)
1 tablespoon milk or soy milk

Beat shortening and sugar together until creamy. Add eggs one at a time, beating after each one. Add vanilla and milk. Beat in oat mix and caraway. Drop on baking sheets with teaspoon 2 inches apart. Bake in preheated oven at 350°F for 12 to 15 minutes. Nuts or coconut may be substituted for caraway seeds.

VARIETY COOKIES

2 1/2 cups Ener-G™ Potato Mix
1 cup brown sugar (packed)
1/2 cup margarine
2 eggs or egg substitute
1 teaspoon vanilla

Cream brown sugar and margarine. Beat in eggs, vanilla and 1 cup potato mix. When batter is too stiff for beater, stir in remaining potato mix. Drop by teaspoonfuls, 2 inches apart, on baking sheet. Bake at 350°F degrees 12 to 15 minutes. For variety, place about 3/4 cup of batter in small bowl. Stir in raisins, nuts, coconut, candied cherries, chopped dates, chocolate chips, peanut butter, etc.

TAIGLACH

1 tablespoon sugar
2 cups flour or flour mix
1 tablespoon oil

3 eggs or egg substitute
2 tablespoons boiling water
1 teaspoon ground almonds (optional)
1 cup honey
1 cup sugar
2 teapoons ginger
1/2 cup nuts (filberts, almonds, soy nuts etc., optional)

Beat the eggs, (or substitute) and 1 tablespoon sugar until thick. Add oil, beating, and then the flour, and almonds if used. Roll into 3 ropes, using more flour if necessary. Cut the ropes into 1/2 inch pieces and roll each piece into a ball. Place on an ungreased baking sheet and bake at 350°F until light brown. Mix honey, sugar and ginger in a saucepan, and bring to a boil. Add the cooked dough, several pieces at a time, and cook until thoroughly coated (about 3 minutes). Stir constantly to avoid burning. Add nuts, if used. Pour small amounts of the mixture into greased muffin tins and cool. Store in the refrigerator.

CAKES

APPLE UPSIDE-DOWN CAKE

2 1/2 cups green apples, peeled and sliced
1/3 cup honey (acceptable kind)
Juice and grated rind of 1 lemon
1/8 teaspoon nutmeg, if allowed
2 tablespoons margarine
1 tablespoon rice flour
Ener-G™ batter for 1 layer yellow cake (See recipe on box.)

Mix the nutmeg, lemon rind, and juice, honey, and tablespoon flour, and coat the apples. Place the apples around the bottom of a well-greased Pyrex pie plate, and pour the rest of the mixture over them. Dot with 1 tablespoon margarine. Mix the batter and pour over apples. Bake a half hour until top is browned. Allow to cool, and turn out onto a plate before the honey-mixture becomes hard.

CHOCOLATE CAKE

3 cups Ener-G™ Oat Mix
1 cup sugar
2 large eggs or egg substitute
1/4 cup margarine
1 1/2 cups milk or soy milk
1 ounce powdered chocolate
1 teaspoon vanilla

Cream together margarine and sugar. Add eggs one at a time and beat. Add vanilla, chocolate, milk and oat mix. Beat until smooth. Pour into 2 round cake pans. Bake in preheated oven at 350°F for 40 to 45 minutes.

POTATO MIX CHOCOLATE CAKE

2 1/2 cups Ener-G™ Potato Mix
4 eggs (separated)
1 1/3 cups granulated sugar
1/4 cup vegetable oil
1 ounce powdered chocolate or carob
1 cup milk
1 teaspoon vanilla

Beat egg whites and set aside. In large bowl beat egg yolks; add sugar gradually while beating. Add oil, chocolate (carob) and vanilla. Alternately beat in milk and potato mix. Gently fold egg whites into batter. Pour into angel food pan. Bake at 350°F for 45 minutes. Turn pan upside down to let cake cook about 2 hours.

HONEY CAKE

1 1/3 cups honey
1/2 cup strong coffee
3 1/2 cups mixed flour or rice flour (see recipe)
2 teaspoons baking powder
1 teaspoon baking soda
1/2 teaspoon cinnamon (optional)
2 teaspoons nutmeg (optional)
4 eggs or egg substitute

2 tablespoons oil
1 cup sugar

Bring the honey to a boil and add coffee. Cool. Sift the flour and spices and baking soda and powder together. Beat the eggs until thick, and add the oil, still beating. Add the sugar, and beat until light yellow. Mix the ingredients gradually, and pour into 2 greased, wax-paper lined loaf pans (bottom only). Bake at 325°F for 1 hour, or until done. Cool.

SHAKER JELLY ROLL CAKE

3 beaten eggs
1 cup sugar
1 cup flour
1 teaspoon baking powder
1/2 teaspoon salt
Jelly to cover

Add to the beaten eggs, sugar and mixture of sifted flour and baking powder with salt. Bake in a large pan for 12 minutes at 350°F. Turn out onto a towel, and spread with jelly. Roll up and wrap in the towel until cool. Sprinkle with sugar if desired.

MARBLE CAKE

2 cups Ener-G™ Oat Mix
1/2 cup cold water
1 ounce chocolate or carob
4 eggs (separated) or egg substitute
1 1/2 cups sugar
1 teaspoon vanilla

Beat egg whites and set aside. Beat egg yolks adding water gradually. Beat until peaks form. Add sugar and vanilla. Beat in oat mix. Fold in egg whites. Divide batter into two bowls. To one bowl add 1 ounce melted baking chocolate and fold. In angel food pan pour part of one batter and part of the other batter. Continue until both batters are used. Place in preheated oven at 350°F for 60 minutes (if you prefer chocolate throughout the cake, add chocolate to batter before folding in egg white).

OAT SPICE CAKE

2 1/2 cups Ener-G™ Oat Mix
1 teaspoon allspice
1 teaspoon ginger
1 teaspoon cinnamon
1/2 cup margarine
1 cup brown sugar
1/4 cup granulated sugar
2 large eggs or egg substitute
1 teaspoon vanilla
1 cup buttermilk

Stir together oat mix and spices. In separate large bowl mix sugar, brown sugar and margarine. Add whole eggs and vanilla. Beat until creamy. Alternately beat in buttermilk and oat mix mixture. Pour into 9" x 9" x 2" pan. Bake in pre-heated oven at 350°F for 50 to 60 minutes.

SPONGE CAKE (No Grain)

8 eggs
1 1/2 cups fine sugar
3 tablespoons lemon juice
1 1/2 teaspoons grated lemon rind
3/4 cup potato starch
Pinch of salt

Separate the eggs into 2 bowls. In an electric mixer, beat the egg yolks for 2 minutes until they are light. Add the lemon rind, juice, and sugar. Mix for 2 more minutes at medium speed with the potato starch added. In the second bowl, beat the egg whites until they are stiff. Fold the egg whites into the egg yolk mixture. Put into a greased tube pan and bake at 350°F for 60 minutes or until the cake springs back when touched. Cool before removing from the pan.

SOYA CAROB CUPCAKES* EMM (Wheat-Free)

1/2 cup brown sugar
1/4 cup oil

2 eggs, separated and beaten
1/3 cup milk
1 cup soya flour
1 teaspoon baking powder
2 tablespoons carob powder
1 teaspoon vanilla

Thoroughly cream oil and sugar; add beaten egg yolks. Add flour and baking powder alternately with liquid to mixture. Then add beaten egg whites, carob and flavoring. Bake at 350°F until done.

SOYA CAKE* EMM (Wheat-Free)

3 cups soya flour
3 teaspoons baking powder
1/2 cup brown sugar
3 drops almond extract
1/2 teaspoon lemon extract
1/3 cup orange juice
1/2 teaspoon vanilla extract
4 eggs, well beaten
1/3 teaspoon baking soda
1/2 teaspoon salt
1 cup cream
1 cup milk (approximately)

Sift dry ingredients together except sugar and soda which are to be rubbed smooth with the eggs. Add to the egg mixture the orange juice and the extracts, then milk and cream. Add the sifted ingredients. Bake at about 350°F for about 45 minutes.

POTATO MIX SPICE CAKE

2 cups Ener-G™ Potato Mix
3/4 teaspoon baking soda
3/4 teaspoon cloves
3/4 teaspoon cinnamon
3/4 teaspoon allspice
1/2 cup shortening
2/3 cup brown sugar (packed)
3/4 cup granulated sugar

2 eggs (unbeaten) or egg substitute
1 cup buttermilk
1 teaspoon vanilla

Mix potato mix, soda and spices together. Set aside. Cream shortening thoroughly and gradually add sugars and cream together. Add eggs one at a time, beating well after each. Add potato mix alternately with buttermilk. Beat after each addition until smooth. Add vanilla and pour batter into two 8" layer pans which have been lined on the bottom with waxed paper. Bake at 350°F for 30 minutes.

RICE POLISH AND RICE FLOUR LEMON CAKE

1 3/4 cups Ener-G™ Rice Polish (sift once before measuring)
1 cup Jolly Joan Rice flour
1 teaspoon baking soda
1 teaspoon salt
1 1/2 cups brown sugar (packed)
1/2 cup soft margarine
2 large unbeaten eggs or egg substitute
1 1/4 cup milk
1 teaspoon lemon extract

Sift all dry ingredients together at least 3 times and set aside. Cream brown sugar and margarine together. Beat in eggs, then lemon extract. Alternately beat in flour mixture and milk until smooth. Oil and dust two 8" cake pans and bake at 350°F for 30 minutes.

RICE POLISH LUXURY CAKE

4 cups sifted Ener-G™ Rice Polish
2 tablespoons double acting baking powder
2 beaten eggs or egg substitute
1/2 cup vegetable oil
1 cup raisins, currants or chopped nuts
1 1/2 cups sugar
1 1/2 teaspoons salt
1 1/2 cups milk
1 teaspoon vanilla

Oil and dust with rice flour or polish two 8" cake pans. Sift Ener-G™ Rice Polish, sugar baking powder and salt together. Add milk, vegetable oil, vanilla and beaten eggs. Beat until smooth. Sprinkle about 1 teaspoon sugar over raisins (just to dust them). Then stir into batter. Pour into cake pans. Bake at 350°F for 30 to 40 minutes.

SPICE CAKE

2 cups flour (or flour mix)
1 cup coffee
1 cup raisins (optional)
1 cup brown sugar
2 eggs or egg substitute
2 tablespoons shortening
1 teaspoon baking soda
1/2 teaspoon salt
1 teaspoon nutmeg
1 teaspoon mace
1 teaspoon cloves, powdered

Heat the coffee, sugar, shortening and raisins. Add the other ingredients and mix. Bake in loaf pan at 350°F until done (about a half hour).

BROWN SUGAR CAKE

2 cups Ener-G™ Potato Mix
1 1/3 cups brown sugar (packed)
2 eggs or egg substitute
1/2 cup margarine
1/2 cup milk
1 teaspoon vanilla

Cream brown sugar and margarine together. Add eggs and beat until creamy. Stir in milk and vanilla, then potato mix. Beat batter until smooth, pour in 2 cake pans. Bake at 350°F for 35 minutes. Cool 5 minutes in pans before removing to cake rack.

WINDTORTE

Shell:
8 egg whites
1/2 teaspoon cream of tartar
2 1/2 cups superfine sugar

Filling:
1/2 pint heavy cream (or soy whipping cream)
2 tablespoons sugar
1/4 cup cognac
3 cups berries (blueberries or raspberries)

Decoration:
4 egg whites
1/4 teaspoon cream of tartar
1 1/2 cups superfine sugar

Heat the oven to 200°F. Butter and flour 2 baking sheets, and remove the excess flour. Outline on each sheet 2 eight inch circles to guide you in making the shell of the cake. Beat the 8 egg whites and cream of tartar until stiff, adding 2 1/4 cups of the sugar when they begin to foam, and the rest of the sugar when stiff. Using a #8 plain tipped pastry tube, pipe the meringue just inside the 3 rings. Bake in slow oven until dry, and cool. To form the bottom (and top, if you wish) pipe the meringue in a spiral around the inside of the ring, until the spiral closes in the middle, and bake. Whip the cream until it begins to thicken and gradually add the sugar, beating constantly. When the cream holds its shape, add the cognac, and then fold in the berries. Spoon into the shell of the cake. If you wish to top, put the layer on top of this. *Note:* The decoration should be done before the filling is added as it must bake 20 minutes.

EGG-FREE DOUBLE LAYER CAKE

5 teaspoons Ener-G™ Egg Replacer (packed)
4 tablespoons water (stir these two ingredients until smooth)
2 1/2 cups sifted cake flour
1 1/2 cups sugar
3 teaspoons baking powder
1 teaspoon salt

1/2 cup soft shortening
1 cup water
1 teaspoon vanilla

Sift flour, sugar, baking powder and salt together. Drop shortening into flour mixture. Drop shortening into flour mixture. Add 3/4 cup water, vanilla and egg replacer. Beat 3 or 4 minutes. Add remaining water and beat 3 minutes. Pour into 8 inch cake pans. Bake in preheated oven at 375°F for 30 to 35 minutes.

EGG-FREE WHITE CAKE WITH SUGAR

4 teaspoons Ener-G™ Egg Replacer
8 tablespoons water
1/3 cup sugar
1/3 cup oil
1 cup milk or soy milk
1 teaspoon vanilla
2 1/2 cups Ener-G™ Rice Mix

Beat the egg replacer and water together to soft peaks. In a separate bowl mix together sugar, oil, milk, and vanilla. Beat in Rice Mix until smooth. Fold in whipped egg replacer until well blended. Pour into two 8" diameter cake pans. Bake at 350°F for 35 minutes.

CANDY

APPLE CANDY II

2 tablespoons unflavored gelatin or agar-agar
1/2 cup cider applesauce, cold
3/4 cup hot applesauce
2 cups sugar, or a bit less, to taste
1 tablespoon vanilla
Powdered sugar

Soak gelatin in the cold applesauce for 10 minutes. Add this mixture to the mixture of hot applesauce and sugar, and simmer for 15 minutes, stirring. Add vanilla and put into a greased 9 inch square pan. Cool, and allow to set. Cut and roll in sugar.

APRICOT OR PEACH CANDY

1 pound of apricots
1/2 cup sugar

Combine the ingredients in a heavy pot and simmer until it is fairly dry. Be careful that it doesn't burn. Blend or process until it is a paste. Spread thin on a sheet of plastic wrap and dry. It can then be rolled, as leather, or cut into shapes with cookie cutters and coated with sugar.

COFFEE GELATIN CANDY

2 tablespoons unflavored gelatin
1 1/2 cups sugar
1 pinch salt
1 1/4 cups very strong hot coffee
1 teaspoon vanilla extract
1/2 cup chopped nuts (unsalted)

Dissolve the gelatin, sugar, and salt in a saucepan, with the coffee. Simmer for about 20 minutes. Allow to cool, and when mixture thickens add the vanilla and the chopped nuts. Allow to set in a pan at room temperature for several hours.

CANDIED NUTS

Small amount of oil
Peanuts
Pumpkin seeds
Sunflower seeds
Sesame seeds
Honey or pure maple syrup
Nut meats (any kind)

Heat a heavy pan on medium heat. Add oil to barely coat bottom of pan. Add the peanuts and the seeds, and roast lightly. Add the nut meats. Remove from heat, and add just enough honey or maple syrup to coat the nuts and seeds.

PROTEIN HALVAH

1 cup sesame seeds
1/4 cup honey
Pinch of salt
6 tablespoons soy protein isolate
1 teaspoon lemon juice (or more to taste)

Heat the sesame seeds in a heavy iron skillet until they begin to brown slightly. Stir constantly. Remove from the hot pan. Puree the sesame seeds in a blender to make a rough paste. Remove the sesame paste and place in a bowl. Stir or knead in the remaining ingredients. Pat out mixture on waxed paper. Chill. Cut into whatever shape and size you fancy.

MARSHMALLOWS II

1 tablespoon unflavored gelatin or agar-agar
1/3 cup water
1 teaspoon vanilla
2/3 cup cane sugar syrup
1/2 cup sugar
Confectioner's sugar or coconut

Boil the water and add sugar and gelatin. Stir until dissolved. Add syrup and vanilla. Beat at high speed until the mixture is quite thick. Cool. Cut in squares. Roll in confectioner's sugar (this contains 3% cornstarch) or coconut.

SWEET SPREADS

SHAKER APPLE BUTTER

3 pounds green apples
1/2 gallon boiled cider (from 1 gallon fresh)
1/2 tablespoon allspice

Cut up the apples, leaving skin on. Bring apples and cider to a boil, and simmer, stirring frequently. When the apples are done, strain through a colander. Cook down until thickened, and add the allspice. Pour into sterile jars and seal.

APPLE JELLY

8 pounds tart apples
4 cups water
Sugar

Wash, core and slice the apples without peeling and place apples and water in a large pot. Bring to a boil and simmer for 20 minutes or until soft. Allow to drip through a jelly bag. Add 3/4 cup of sugar for every cup of juice and boil for 20 minutes. Remove scum that forms. Pour into sterilized jars and follow canning directions.

BEET PRESERVES

2 pounds beets
2 cups sugar
2 cups honey
1 tablespoon ginger
3 small sliced lemons

Cook the beets until tender in water to cover. Drain. Remove the skins and cut into very small chunks. Combine the honey, sugar, ginger, and lemons in a saucepan and bring to a boil. Add the beets, and simmer, stirring occasionally, for 3/4 of an hour, until beets are translucent. Put into sterilized hot jars, and seal.

CRANBERRY JELLY

4 quarts cranberries
2 quarts water
8 cups sugar

In a large heavy pot, bring the berries and the water to a boil. Lower the heat to medium, and cook until the berries pop open (15 minutes). Strain through a jelly bag, and add the sugar. Boil until the mixture reaches the jelling point. Pour into sterilized jars and seal.

CRANBERRY SAUCE

2 cups cranberries, washed
2 cups boiling water
2 cups sugar

Put the cranberries and water in a large pot and simmer until they are done (berries will break open). Force through a sieve and put in the pot again, adding sugar. Simmer until thickened. Pour into a mold if desired, and chill.

RED CURRANT JELLY

2 pounds red currants
1 cup water
2 cups sugar

Simmer the currants in the water until the skins break. Hang in a jelly bag and allow juice to drip through into a bowl. Measure the juice into a pan, and for each pint of juice add 2 cups sugar. Stir until dissolved and boil until jelling point is reached.

CURRANT PRESERVES

2 pounds currants
1 1/2 pounds sugar

Mash the currants and put in a pot. Simmer for 15 minutes and add the sugar, stirring. Boil for 2 minutes, place in sterilized jars and seal.

GUAVA JELLY

2 pounds guava pulp
1 cup water
Sugar
Juice of 2 limes

Use slightly underripe guavas and wash, prick with a fork and simmer until soft. Put pulp in a jelly bag and allow to drip through. Add 2 cups of sugar for each 2 cups of juice. Heat to dissolve sugar, stirring. Add the lime juice and cook until jelling point is reached. Place in sterilized jars and seal.

PEAR HONEY

1 cup water
6 cups sugar
12 pears
2 cloves in spice bag

Peel and core pears. Boil water and sugar together until slightly thickened. Add pears and simmer for 1 hour. Stir during this time to avoid burning. Add cloves for last 1/2 hour. Remove, pour into sterilized jars, and follow canning directions for the size of the jars used.

SHAKER DAMSON PLUM "CHEESE"

2 pounds plums
Water to cover
Sugar in ratio of 1/2 cup to 2 cups pulp

Boil the plums in water to cover and force the pulp through a sieve. Add the sugar and boil until it begins to stick to the sides. Pour into sterile jars and seal.

POMEGRANATE JELLY

4 cups pomegranate juice
7 1/2 cups sugar
3 tablespoons lemon juice
1 bottle liquid pectin

Juice the pomegranates (be careful, they stain). Mix the juice, lemon juice and sugar, and bring to a boil in a large pot. Add the pectin, and follow the directions on bottle – or boil for 30 seconds, stirring, remove from heat, skim, put into sterile jars and seal.

ROSE FRUIT JAM

2 cups rose hips
1 cup water
2 cups sugar

Place the water and fruit in a pan and simmer until the rose hips are soft. To each two cups of strained pulp, add the given amount of sugar, and simmer until thick. Put into sterilized jars and follow canning directions for the size of the jars.

SWEET SAUCES AND SYRUPS

APRICOT SAUCE

1 pound fresh apricots
1 teaspoon lemon juice (or 1/4 teaspoon ascorbic acid)
1/2 cup sugar
Pinch salt

Process all the ingredients until purees. Force through a sieve.

APRICOT SAUCE II

3/4 cup apricot jam
1/2 cup water
1 tablespoon sugar
1 tablespoon kirsh (or 2 tablespoons lemon juice)

Puree the jam and put in a small sauce-pan, along with the sugar and water. Simmer until thickened, and if desired, add the kirsh or a bit of lemon juice (to taste). Use as a dessert sauce.

SHAKER RASPBERRY SAUCE

2 cups raspberries, washed
1 cup water
1 cup sugar
1/2 cup currant jelly

Cook the raspberries in water for 20 minutes at medium-low heat. If you wish a clear syrup, allow to drip through a jelly-bag, otherwise, force through a strainer. Add the jelly and sugar to this and simmer until the sauce is thick. Chill.

BLUEBERRY SYRUP

3 cups blueberries
3/4 cup sugar
3/4 cup water
1 teaspoon lemon juice (or 1/2 teaspoon ascorbic acid)

Wash berries and place all ingredients in a heavy pot. Simmer until mixture has become "syrupy."

CRANBERRY SYRUP

1 quart Ocean Spray ™ fresh cranberries
2 cups water
1 cup sugar

Wash fruit carefully and drain. Trasnfer berries to a medium saucepan. Add the water and heat to boiling. Reduce heat and simmer for 10 minutes. Strain through cheesecloth to get the maximum amout of liquid. Measure the juice and for each cup of juice, add 1 cup sugar. Cook over medium heat, stirring until the sugar is dissolved and it has come to a boil. Boil for 2 minutes, and remove from heat. Skim off any froth and pour into sterilized jars and seal. (This recipe was provided by Ocean Spray™.)

PLUM, CURRANT OR BERRY SYRUP

Fruit
Water
Sugar

Cook the cleaned fruit in a tiny bit of water. Press to extract the juice from cooked fruit, and then pour into a jelly bag. If you wish clear syrup, allow the juice to drip out. Otherwise, you can use 2 1/2 cups of juice and bring to a boil, stirring. Put in bottles, and seal.

COFFEE SYRUP

1/3 cup strong coffee
1/2 cup sugar

Simmer the two ingredients in pot until slightly thickened.

REFERENCE MATERIALS
COOKING TIPS

Rice Flour (Glutinous):
Recipes made with "sweet-rice flour" (glutinous rice flour) can be frozen and reheated. While this flour holds together, it does not contain gluten.

Cider Sweetener (Shaker):
Boil down 4 gallons of cider until only 1 gallon is left. This syrup may be used to sweeten applesauce, pies, or as a sugar substitute.

Date Sugar:
Date sugar is made by grinding very dry dates into a powder (or as fine as possible). The metal blade in your food processor may be used for this. If your children are sensitive to cornstarch, be alert if you buy cut dates, as they are often coated with cornstarch to prevent sticking.

Powdered Sugar:
To avoid the 3% cornstarch present in confectioners sugar, grind granulated sugar in a food processor. It takes a while, but does produce a fine powder. Use the metal blade.

Thickeners:
Many stir-fry recipes require cornstarch for thickening the sauce. To avoid this, dissolve 1 tablespoon arrowroot flour in 1/4 cup water or broth. Add this to the liquid, and boil for a short time.

Soy Sauce Substitute:
If you cannot use soy sauce because of the soy, wheat or corn content, add a small amount of salt at the end of the cooking period.

HOME PREPARATION OF BASIC SUPPLIES

To avoid the additives and other problems associated with processed foods, the most practical solution is to process your own. With the growing popularity of home canning and freezing, it is once again easy to find the necessary tools; jars, lids and other supplies.

Once you have discovered which fruits and vegetables are permitted in your diet, find out the season in which they are most plentiful. The Department of Agriculture in most states maintains a " Farmer to Consumer" list of local farmers who sell their products directly to the consumer (generally at much lower prices than the major chains). Farmers' markets are also good sources of produce, as are some health food stores, if you need unsprayed produce. Be sure to check the sources, however, as not all food labeled "natural" or "organic" is free of pesticides. The definition of these two terms is still under debate.

Both the BALL™ and KERR™ companies issue canning guides which are available for nominal sums. Coupons and addresses are usually on the jar-lid packages. Many "basic" cookbooks include canning and freezing guides.

To provide variety, look up all the possible ways of preparing the acceptable foods. For example, apricots can be stewed, spiced, dried, made into apricot "leather," jams or preserves, or frozen for later use in pies, tarts and recipes. If you freeze some of the fruit for pies, freezing it in pie tins mixed with the sugar and tapioca (or other thickener) will provide you with your own "convenience foods."

Canning fruit requires simple, inexpensive equipment – a water bath canner (a very large pot with a cover and a rack so the cans don't bounce around and break), jars and self-sealing caps.

If you can take advantage of solar drying, a drying rack is very easy to build. You will need a box-shape made of four 1' x 3' boards, a coated screen floor and top, and four small blocks for legs (to aid in air circulation). (See picture on following page.) An electric food drier is preferable if the weather in your area is variable or if you are allergic to molds which might land on food in a solar drying rack. Prices vary according to the capabilities of the machine.

181

Fruits may be sulphured to avoid discoloration, although this is not necessary. If you are sensitive to sulfites (usually used in sulferization), dipping the fruit in ascorbic acid (Vitamin C) solution before drying will also minimize discoloration. Fruit can also be dried with no processing, although it will appear quite dark when dry.

Some fruits (prunes, for example) need to be blanched or pierced before drying as the skins are tough. Blanching can be avoided by halving the fruit or cutting it into sections. (It will also dry more quickly this way.)

Be sure the fruit is not injured and contains no mold before you process or dry it. This will eliminate problems during storage.

Special treats can be made from the leftovers of home processing. From extra fruit puree, you can make fruit "leather" or fruit "chews" (the "leather" by spreading on plastic wrap and drying, and the "chews" by adding chopped nuts or dry soybeans, spreading, drying, and cutting into pieces). Extra syrup of stewed fruit can be boiled down to make fruit syrups for use on pancakes and waffles or in flavored drinks. Fruit syrups must be processed like canned fruit to keep them for later use. Very fine purees can be processed and diluted as fruit drinks, and adding ascorbic acid (usually 1 teaspoon per quart – see instructions on package) makes these a good substitute for orange juice in the morning.

Vegetables can also be canned and dried, although canning non-acidic items requires a pressurized canner. Dried vegetables can be ground up and mixed for use as "instant" soups, or used sliced, as "chips" for dips. They can also be used in stews.

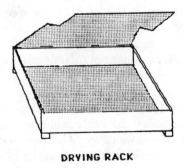

DRYING RACK

Freezing allows vegetables and fruit to retain better flavor, than canning or drying, and additive-free frozen vegetables are readily available. Freezing has the additional advantage of preventing the growth of yeasts and mold during storage. There are some things you need to consider when choosing a method of preserving food: the length of time you wish to keep the food (dried and canned foods have longer shelf-life than frozen), the use to which you will put the finished product, and whether the food (with additions, if necessary) will provide the allergic child with the nutrition he/she needs.

Bibliography for Food Preservation

The following are both extensive booklets containing methods, recipes and problem-solving sections.

Kerr Home Canning and Freezing Book available from Kerr Glass Manufacturing Corporation, Consumer Products Division Sand Springs, OK or in stores which carry Kerr jars and caps.

Ball Blue Book – Easy Guide to Tasty, Thrifty Canning and Freezing from Ball Corporation, Muncie, IN or in stores which carry Ball jars and caps.

The following books, plus pamphlets from your State University Agricultural Extension, will be helpful:

Rombauer, Irma S. and Marion Rombauer Becker. *The Joy of Cooking.* Indianapolis: Bobbs-Merrill Co., Inc., 1964.

The Settlement Book Co.: *The Settlement Cook Book.* New York: Simon and Shuster, 1976.

NUTRIENT TABLES AND FOOD FAMILIES

It is important when you are dealing with growing children to be certain their diet is not lacking in nutrients. If your child is following an extremely restricted diet, discussion with a dietician or nutritionist is helpful.

If you own a computer, there are a variety of available programs which can help you evaluate your child's diet on a continuing basis. Two of these are The Dietician from Dietware and The Nutritionist. Most of these programs should be used with the *Department of Agriculture Handbook #8–Composition of Foods* for a more complete evaluation of the nutrition provided by the diet, but this should not take the place of primary consultation with a qualified practitioner.

The Dietician, for example, contains a list of 700 foods, and allows the user to add more foods to the existing list. The program provides information on (and complete totals of) calories, carbohydrates, proteins, fats, cholesterol and sodium. You can enter individual foods or quantities used for recipes. Allowances are made for variable cooking methods (boiled, broiled, fried, etc.) and condition (lean, fat). The results can be stored and/or printed. These programs provide a good method of planning and reviewing nutritional intake.

(See Bibliography for further information.)

Many new nutrition education programs are being published, and parents are well-advised to read all they can about nutrition. The U.S. Government Publications Office has a list of available free booklets, and your public library is also a good source.

FOOD FAMILIES

Plants

Apple
    apple
    apple cider
    crabapple
    pectin

Arum
    dasheen
    poi
    taro

Beech
    beechnut
    chestnut

Borage
    borage

Buckwheat
    buckwheat
    rhubarb
    sorrel

Cashew
    cashew
    mango
    pistachio

Citrus
    angostura
    citron
    grapefruit
    kumquat
    lemon
    lime
    orange

Arrowroot
    arrowroot

Banana
    banana
    plantain

Birch
    filbert
    hazelnut

Brazil nut
    brazil nut

Cactus
    cactus
    prickly pear

Chicory
    chicory

Cochliospernum
    gum guaiac
    karaya gum

quince
tangelo
tangerine

Composite
artichoke
chicory
dandelion
endive
escarole
jerusalem artichoke
lettuce (head &leaf)
salsify
sunflower
sesame
pyrethrum

Ebony
persimmon

Fungus
mushroom
yeast

Ginger
cardamom
ginger
tumeric

Gooseberry
currant
gooseberry

Goosefoot
beet (including
  sugar beet)
chard
spinach
thistle

Gourd
casaba
cantaloupe
cucumber
chayote
honeydew
muskmelon
Persian melon
pumpkin
squash(summer & winter)
water melon

Grape
grape(European &
  American)

Heath
    blueberry
    cranberry
    huckleberry
    lingonberry
    wintergreen

Honeysuckle
    elderberry

Laurel
    avocado
    bay leaves
    cinnamon
    sassafrass

Holly
    yerba mate

Iris
    saffron

Legume
    black-eyed peas
    carob
    (St. John's bread)
    chick pea
    (garbanzo)
    fenugreek
    field pea
    green pea
    guar gum
    gum acacia
    gum tragacanth
    jack bean
    kidney bean
    lentil
    licorice
    lima bean
    mung bean
    navy bean
    peanut
    pinto bean
    soybean
    string bean
    tamarind
    tonka bean
    white bean
    wax bean

Lily
asparagus
chives
garlic
leek
onion
sarsaparilla
shallots

Mallow
maple
cottonseed
okra

Morning Glory
sweet potato

Mustard
broccoli
brussel sprouts
cabbage
cauliflower
celery
Chinese cabbage
collard
kale
kohlrabi
horseradish
mustard
mustard greens

Madder
coffee

Mint
basil
horehound
marjoram
mint
oregano
peppermint
rosemary
savory
spearmint
thyme

Mulberry
fig
hop
mulberry

Myrtle
allspice
bayberry
clove
eucalytus
guava

188

radishes
rutabaga
turnips
watercress

Nightshade
bell pepper
chili pepper
cayenne
eggplant
ground cherry
paprika
potato (white)
tomato

Nutmeg
mace
nutmeg

Oak
chestnut

Olive
jasmine
olive

Orchid
vanilla

Palm
coconut
date
sago

Papaw
papaya

Parsley
angelica
anise
caraway
carrots
celeriac
celery
chervil
coriander
cumin
dill
fennel
lovage
parsley
parsnips

star anise

Pepper
black pepper
white pepper

Pineapple
pineapple

Pomegranate
pomegranate

Rose
blackberry
boysenberry
dewberry
hackberry
loganberry
raspberry
strawberry
youngberry

Soapberry
lichi nut

Spurge
tapioca

Pine
juniper
pinion nut

Plum
apricot
almond
cherry
nectarine
peach
plum
prune

Poppy
poppy seed

Sapodillo
chickle
sapodillo

Stercula
cocoa
cola

Walnut
black walnut
butternut
English walnut
hickory
pecan

Water Chestnut
    water chestnut

Animals

Amphibians
    frog

Cephalopods
    octopus
    squid

Fish
    anchovy
    bluefish
    bonito, tuna, mackerel
    bullhead, catfish
    butterfish
    carp
    chub
    cod
    eel
    flounder
    haddock
    hake
    halibut
    herring
    mullet
    perch

Yam
    Chinese potato
    yam

Birds
    chicken
    duck
    goose
    grouse
    guinea hen
    partridge
    pheasant
    turkey
    eggs

Crustaceans
    crab
    crayfish
    lobster
    prawn
    shrimp

Gastropods
    abalone
    snail

pickerel
pike
pollock
red snapper, porgy
roach
sailfish
salmon, trout
smelt
sole
sturgeon
sunfish
tarpon
white bass, rockfish

Mammals
beef, veal
cow's milk
dairy products
goat
mutton or lamb
pork
rabbit
squirrel
venison

Reptiles
rattlesnake
turtle

Mollusks
clam
mussel
oyster
scallop
squid

NUTRIENT TABLES

The following charts were compiled from the *United States Department of Agriculture Handbook #8, Composition of Foods*, and several plant and animal classification lists. Those numbers in parentheses indicate that the values are computed from another form of the food or from a similar food. Unless otherwise noted, all food was considered in its raw state. Cooking may change the values somewhat.

Food	Family	Relatives or Products	Calories	Protein (Grams)	Carbo-hydrates	Calcium
Apple	apple crabapple	cider, pectin	50–60	.2	14.5	7
Apricot	plum	almond, cherry, nectarine, peach, plum, prune	51	1.0	12.8	17
Artichoke	composite	Jerusalem artichoke, camomile, endive, escarole, lettuce, safflower, salsify, sunflower, tarragon, yarrow, wormwood, ragweed	9–40	2.9	10.6	51
Asparagus	lily	chives, aloes, garlic, leek, onion, sarsaparilla, shallot	26	2.5	5.0	22
Avocados	laurel	bay leaf, camphor, cinnamon, laurel, sassafras	167	2.1	6.3	10
Bacon, cured	mammal	pork, (in any form)	665	8.4	1.0	13
Bacon, Canadian	mammal	pork, (in any form)	216	20.0	.3	12
Bamboo Shoots	grain corn, oat, rice,	barley, ale, lager cane rye, sorghum, wheat, pumpernickle	27	2.6	5.2	13
Bananas	banana	manila, hemp	85	1.1	22.2	8
Barley, pearl	grain	(see bamboo shoots)	349	8.2	78.8	16
Bass, black sea	fish, ocean	perch, red mullet	93	19.2	0	
smallmouth	fish, freshwater		104	18.9	0	
Beans, common mature white	legume	acacia, arabic, kidney bean, green bean, lima bean, navy bean, soy bean, wax bean, locust bean, carob, cassia, fenugreek	340	22.3	61.3	144
Beans, snap	legume	(see common white)	32	1.9	7.1	56
yellow, wax	legume	(see common white)	27	1.7	6.0	56
Beef, choice	mammal	antelope, buffalo, goat, sheep	301	17.4	0	10
Blackberries	rose	raspberry, loganberry, strawberry	58	1.2	12.9	32

Phosphorus milligrams	Iron milligrams	Potassium milligrams	Vitamin A international units	Thiamin milligrams	Riboflavin milligrams	Niacin milligrams	Ascorbic Acid milligrams
10	.3	110	90	.03	.02	.1	4
23	.5	281	2700	.03	.04	.6	10
88	1.3	430	160	.08	.05	1.0	12
62	1.0	278	900	.18	.20	1.5	33
42	.6	604	290	.11	.20	1.6	14
108	1.2	130		36	.11	1.8	
180	3.0	392		.83	.22	4.7	
59	.5	533	20	.15	.07	.6	4
26	.7	370	190	.05	.06	.7	10
189	2.0	160		.12	.05	3.1	
		256					
192				.10	.03	2.1	
425	7.8	1,196		.65	.22	2.4	
44	.8	243	600	.08	.11	.5	19
43	.8	243	250	.08	.11	.5	20
161	2.6	370	50	.07	.17	4.2	
19	.9	170	200	.03	.04	.4	21

Food	Family	Relatives or Products	Calories	Protein (Grams)	Carbo-hydrates	Calcium
Blueberries	heath	cranberry, huckle-berry, wintergreen, lingonberry	62	7	15.3	15
Broccoli	mustard	mustard, cabbage, cauli-flower, brussel sprouts, turnips, collard, rutaba-gas, kale, kohlrabi, celery cabbage, radish, horse-radish, watercress	32	3.6	5.9	103
Buckwheat	buckwheat	rhubarb, sorrel	335	11.7	72.9	114
Cabbage	mustard	(see broccoli)	24	1.3	5.4	49
Cabbage, Chinese	mustard	(see broccoli)	14	1.2	3.0	43
Carob flour	legume	(see beans)	180	4.5	80.7	352
Carrots	parsley	parsley, parsnips, celery, celeriac, caraway, cori-ander, dill, cumin, fennel, angelica, anise	42	1.1	9.7	37
Cashew nuts	cashew	pistachio, mango, poison ivy, poison oak	561	17.2	29.1	38
Cauliflower	mustard	(see broccoli)	27	2.7	5.2	25
Celery	parsley	(see carrots)	17	.9	3.9	39
Chard, Swiss	goosefoot	(see spinach)	25	2.4	4.6	88
Cherries, sweet	plum, apricot, almond, nectarine	plums, peach	70	1.3	17.4	22
Chicken, light	birds	eggs, turkey, duck, goose, squab, pheasant	166	31.6	0	11
dark		grouse, partridge	176	28.0	0	13
Chickpeas (garbanzos)	legume	(see beans)	360	20.5	61.0	150
Coconut meat	palm, cabbage, sago	date, palm	346	3.5	9.4	13
Cod	fish	haddock, whiting, hake, sole, turbot, halibut	170	28.5	0	31
Collards	mustard	(see broccoli)	45	4.8	7.5	250
Corn, sweet	cereal, rye, oats, rice, sorghum, cane, bamboo, millet	wheat, barley	96	3.5	22.1	3

Phosphorus milligrams	Iron milligrams	Potassium milligrams	Vitamin A international units	Thiamin milligrams	Riboflavin milligrams	Niacin milligrams	Ascorbic Acid milligrams
13	1.0	81	100	.03	.06	.5	14
78	1.1	382	2,500	.10	.23	.9	113
282	3.1	448	0	.60	—	4.4	0
29	.4	233	130	.05	.05	.3	47
40	.6	253	150	.05	.04	.6	25
81	—	—	—	—	—	—	—
36	.7	341	11.000	.06	.05	.6	8
373	3.8	464	100	.43	.25	1.8	—
56	1.1	295	60	.11	.10	.7	78
28	.3	341	240	.03	.03	.3	9
39	3.2	550	6,500	.06	.17	.5	32
19	.4	191	110	.05	.06	4	10
265	1.3	411	60	.04	.10	11.6	—
229	1.7	321	150	.07	.23	5.6	—
331	6.9	797	50	.31	.15	2.0	—
95	1.7	256	0	.05	.02	.5	3
274	1.0	407	180	.08	.11	3.0	—
82	1.5	450	9,300	.16	.31	1.7	152
111	.7	280	400	.15	.12	1.7	12

Food	Family	Relatives or Products	Calories	Protein (Grams)	Carbo-hydrates	Calcium
corn flour	(see above)		368	7.8	76.3	6
Cranberries	heath	(see blueberry)	46	4	10.8	14
Currants	heath	(see blueberry)	54	1.7	13.1	60
Duck, domesticated	bird	(see chicken)	326	16	0	10
Eggplant	nightshade	potato, tomato, thorn-apple, tobacco, cayenne pepper, chili pepper	25	1.2	5.6	12
Figs	mulberry	mulberry, breadfruit, hop	80	1.2	20.3	35
Flatfishes	fish	flounder, sole, sandabs	79	16.7	0	12
Ginger root	ginger	arrowroot, turmeric, cardamom	49	1.4	9.5	23
Goose, domesticated	bird	(see chicken)	354	16.4	0	10
Gooseberries	gooseberry	currants, also heath (blueberry)	39	0.8	9.7	18
Grapefruit	citrus	orange, citron, lemon, lime, quince, tangelo, tangerine, kumquat	41	.5	10.6	16
Grapes, European	grape	Malaga, muscat, Thompson, emperor, Tokay	67	.6	17.3	12
American	grape	Concord, Delaware, Niagara, catawba, scuppernong	69	1.3	15.7	16
Guava	myrtle	allspice, clove, roseapple	62	.8	15.0	23
Guinea Hen	bird	(see chicken)	156	23.1	0	—
Haddock	fish	cod, pollock, whiting	79	18.3	0	23
Halibut, Atlantic or Pacific	fish	flounder	100	20.9	0	13
Lamb choice	mammal	(see beef)	263	16.5	0	10
Lemon juice	citrus	(see grapefruit)	25	5	8.0	7
Lentils	legume	(see beans)	340	24.7	60.1	79
Lettuce crisp	composite	endive, escarole, arti-choke, chicory, dande-lion, salsify, sunflower,	13	.9	2.9	20

198

Phosphorus milligrams	Iron milligrams	Potassium milligrams	Vitamin A international units	Thiamin milligrams	Riboflavin milligrams	Niacin milligrams	Ascorbic Acid milligrams
164	1.8	—	340	.20	.06	1.4	0
10	.5	82	40	.03	.02	.1	11
40	1.1	372	230	.05	.05	.3	200
176	1.6	—	—	.08	.19	6.7	—
26	.7	214	10	.05	.05	.6	5
22	.6	194	80	.06	.05	.4	2
195	.8	342	—	.05	.05	1.7	—
36	2.1	264	10	.02	.04	.7	4
176	1.6	—	—	.08	.19	6.7	—
15	.5	155	290	—	—	—	33
16	.4	135	80	.04	.02	.2	38
20	.4	173	100	.05	.03	.3	4
12	.4	158	100	.05	.03	.3	4
42	.9	289	280	.05	.05	1.2	242
—	—	—	—	—	—	—	—
197	.7	304	—	.04	.07	3.0	—
211	.7	449	440	.07	.07	8.3	—
147	1.2	295	—	.15	.20	4.8	—
10	.2	141	20	.03	.01	.1	46
377	6.8	790	60	.37	.22	2.0	—
22	.5	175	330	.06	.06	.3	6

Food	Family	Relatives or Products	Calories	Protein (Grams)	Carbo-hydrates	Calcium
		sesame, absinthe, vermouth, pyrethrum, camomile, tarragon				
Limes	citrus	(see grapefruit)	28	.7	9.5	33
Liver Beef	mammal	(see beef)	140	19.9	5.3	8
Calf		(see beef)	140	19.2	4.1	8
Chicken		(see chicken)	129	19.7	2.9	12
Lamb		(see beef)	136	21	2.9	10
Turkey		(see chicken)	138	21.2	2.9	—
Lobster	crustacea	crayfish, prawn, shrimp	91	16.9	0.5	29
Loquats	apple	crabapple, apple, pear, manzanilla, quince, juneberry	48	.4	12.4	20
Mackerel	fish	bonito, tuna	191	19	0	5
Molasses cane, blackstrap		cane sugar	213	—	55	684
Muskmelons Cantaloupe	gourd	chayote, cucumber, pumpkin, summer squash, winter squash, watermelon, gherkin casaba, honeydew	30	.7	7.5	14
Okra	mallow	cottonseed	36	2.4	7.6	92
Olives	olive	jasmine, manzanilla	129	1.1	2.6	84
Onions	lily	asparagus, chives, leek, sarsaparilla, shallot	38	1.5	8.7	27
Oranges	citrus	(see grapefruit)	49	1.0	12.2	41
Papayas	papaya		39	.6	10.0	20
Parsley	parsley	angelica, anise, (see carrots)	44	3.6	8.5	203
Peaches	plum	(see apricot)	38	.6	9.7	9
Peanuts	legume	(see beans)	564	26	18.6	69
Pears	apple	(see loquats)	61	.7	15.3	8
Peas immature	legume	(see beans)	84	6.3	14.4	26
Peppers, sweet green	nightshade	(see eggplant)	22	1.2	4.8	9

Phosphorus milligrams	Iron milligrams	Potassium milligrams	Vitamin A international units	Thiamin milligrams	Riboflavin milligrams	Niacin milligrams	Ascorbic Acid milligrams
18	.6	102	10	.03	.02	.2	37
352	6.5	281	43,900	.25	3.26	13.6	31
333	8.8	281	22,500	.20	2.72	11.4	36
236	7.9	172	12,100	.19	2.49	10.8	17
349	10.9	202	50,500	.40	3.28	16.9	33
	—	160	17,700	.18	1.93	13.2	—
183	0.6	—	—	.40	.05	1.5	—
36	.4	348	670	—	—	—	1
239	1.0	—	450	.15	.33	8.2	—
84	16.1	2,927	—	.11	.19	2.0	—
16	.4	251	3,400	—	—	—	—
51	.6	249	520	.17	.21	1.0	31
16	1.6	34	60	trace	trace	—	—
36	.5	157	40	.03	.04	.2	10
20	.4	200	200	.10	.04	4	50
16	.3	234	1,700	.04	.04	.3	56
63	6.2	727	8,500	.12	.26	1.2	172
19	.5	202	1,330	.02	.05	1.0	7
401	2.1	674	—	1.14	.13	17.2	0
11	.3	130	20	.02	.04	.1	4
116	1.9	316	640	.35	.14	1.9	27
22	.7	213	420	.08	.08	.5	128

Food	Family	Relatives or Products	Calories	Protein (Grams)	Carbo-hydrates	Calcium
ripe red			31	1.4	7.1	13
Pineapple	pineapple		52	0.4	13.7	17
Plums damson	plum	(see apricot)	66	.5	17.8	18
Popcorn	grain	(see corn)	386	12.7	76.7	11
Pork fresh	mammal	(see beef)	553	9.1	0	5
Potatoes	nightshade	(see eggplant)	76	2.1	17.1	7
Prunes	plum	(see apricot)	344	3.3	91.3	90
Pumpkin	gourd	(see muskmelon)	26	1.0	6.5	21
Pumpkin and Squash seeds	gourd		553	29.0	15.0	51
Quail	bird	(see chicken)	168	25	0	—
Rabbit domesticated	mammal	(see beef)	162	21	0	20
Raisins	grape	(see grape)	289	2.5	77.4	62
Raspberries black	rose	(see blackberry)	73	1.5	15.7	30
red			57	1.2	13.6	22
Red Snapper	fish	porgy	93	19.8	0	16
Reindeer	mammal	(see beef)	127	21.8	0	—
Rhubarb	buckwheat	(see buckwheat)	16	.6	3.7	96
Rice brown	grain	(see corn)	360	7.5	77.4	32
white, enriched			363	6.7	80.4	24
unenriched			363	6.7	80.4	24
glutinous			361	5.6	79.8	36
Rice polish	grain	(see corn)	265	12.1	57.7	69
Rye	grain	(see corn)	334	12.1	73.4	38
Salmon Atlantic	fish	grayling, trout, whitefish	217	22.5	0	79
Pink			119	20	0	—
Scallops	mussel	clam, cockle, oyster	81	15.3	3.3	26
Shrimp	crustacea	crayfish, lobster, prawn	91	18.1	1.5	63

Phosphorus milligrams	Iron milligrams	Potassium milligrams	Vitamin A international units	Thiamin milligrams	Riboflavin milligrams	Niacin milligrams	Ascorbic Acid milligrams
30	.6	—	4,450	.08	.08	.5	204
8	0.5	146	70	.09	.03	.2	17
17	.5	299	300	.08	.03	.5	—
281	2.7	—	—	—	.12	2.2	0
88	1.4	70	0	.44	.10	2.4	—
53	.6	407	trace	.10	.04	1.5	20
107	4.4	940	2,170	.12	.22	2.1	4
44	.8	340	1,600	.05	.11	.6	9
1,144	11.2	—	70	.24	.19	2.4	—
—	—	—	—	—	—	—	—
352	1.3	385	—	.08	.06	12.8	—
101	3.5	763	20	.11	.08	.5	1
22	.9	199	trace	.03	.09	.9	18
22	.9	168	130	.03	.09	.9	25
214	.8	323	—	.17	.02	—	—
—	5.3	—	—	.33	.68	5.5	—
18	.8	251	100	.03	.07	.3	9
221	1.6	214	0	.34	.05	4.7	0
94	2.9	92	0	.44	—	3.5	0
94	.8	92	0	.07	.03	1.6	0
100	2.0	130	0	2.26	.25	29.8	0
1,106	16.1	714	0	1.84	.18	28.2	0
376	3.7	467	0	.43	.22	1.6	0
186	.9	—	—	—	.08	7.2	9
—	—	306	—	.14	.05	—	—
208	1.8	396	—	.06	1.3	—	—
166	1.6	220	—	.02	.03	3.2	—

Food	Family	Relatives or Products	Calories	Protein (Grams)	Carbo-hydrates	Calcium
Soybeans Immature	legume	(see beans)	134	10	13.2	67
Mature			403	34.1	33.5	226
Soybean curd (Tofu)	legume	(see beans)	72	7.8	2.4	128
Spinach	goosefoot	beet, chard, lamb quarters, thistle	26	3.2	4.3	93
Squab	bird	(see chicken)	279	18.6	0	17
Squash Summer	gourd	(see pumpkin)	19	1.1	4.2	28
Winter			50	1.4	12.4	22
Sweet Potatoes	Morning glory		114	1.7	26.3	32
Tangerines	citrus	(see grapefruit)	46	.8	11.6	40
Tapioca	spurge		352	.6	86.4	10
Tomatoes	nightshade	(see eggplant)	22	1.1	4.7	13
Turkey	bird	(see chicken)	218	20.1	0	—
Turnips	mustard	(see broccoli)	30	1.0	6.6	39
Veal	mammal	(see beef)	223	18.5	0	11
Venison	mammal	(see beef)	126	21	0	10
Water chestnut	water chestnut		79	1.4	19	4
Watercress	mustard	(see broccoli)	19	2.2	3.0	151
Watermelon	gourd	(see cantaloupe)	26	.5	6.4	7
Wheat whole grain red spring	grain	(see corn)	330	14	69.1	36
flour (wholewheat)			333	13.3	71	41
all-purpose (enriched)			364	10.5	76.1	16
Wild rice	grain	(see corn)	353	14.1	75.3	19
Yam	yam		101	2.1	23.2	20
Yeast baker's compressed	yeast		86	12.1	11	13

Phosphorus milligrams	Iron milligrams	Potassium milligrams	Vitamin A international units	Thiamin milligrams	Riboflavin milligrams	Niacin milligrams	Ascorbic Acid milligrams
225	2.8	—	690	.44	.16	1.4	29
554	8.4	1,677	80	1.10	.31	2.2	—
126	1.9	42	0	.06	.03	.1	0
51	3.1	470	8,100	.10	.20	.6	51
411	—	—	—	—	—	—	—
29	.4	202	410	.05	.09	1.0	22
38	.6	369	3,700	.05	.11	.6	13
47	.7	243	8,800	.1	.06	.6	21
18	.4	126	420	.06	.02	.1	31
18	.4	18	0	0	0	0	0
27	.5	244	900	.06	.04	.7	23
—	—	—	—	—	—	—	—
30	.5	268	trace	.04	.07	.6	36
185	2.8	320	—	14	.25	6.2	—
249	—	—	—	23	.48	6.3	—
65	6	500	0	.14	.20	1	4
54	1.7	282	4,900	.08	.16	.9	79
10	.5	100	590	.03	.03	.2	7
383	3.1	370	0	.57	.12	4.3	0
372	3.3	370	0	.55	.12	4.3	0
87	2.9	95	0	.44	.26	3.5	0
339	4.2	220	0	.45	.63	6.2	0
69	.6	600	trace	.10	.04	.5	9
394	4.9	610	trace	.71	1.65	11.2	trace

LABELING AND ADDITIVES

There is a section in the FDA Codes entitled "Hypoallergenic Foods." In order for a food to use this designation on the label, the codes state that the label must list:

a) the common name and proportion of each ingredient including spices, flavoring and coloring

b) a qualification of the name of each ingredient which reveals the plant or animal source if it is not clear from the food itself

c) ingredients which might change its allergenic properties

It is not surprising that this label is not seen on grocery store shelves. There are few food processors who would choose to submit to these rules when they could as easily state that the product contains "spices and natural flavorings" instead. Even special infant formulas are listed as "milk free" or "corn free" instead of "hypoallergenic." This does make sense because the mechanisms of food allergy are not completely understood and it seems to be possible for individuals to have an allergic response to virtually any food protein (and, some researchers believe, to a *hapten* – a normally non-allergenic substance which links itself to another, forming a molecule large enough to incite an allergic reaction).

To make labeling easier for the processors, certain ingredients and combinations of ingredients are considered by the FDA to be "standards of identity" for the industry. That is, these ingredients constitute part of the definition of the product. The standard for a given product includes both mandatory and optional ingredients, and a product may contain some or all of these ingredients without listing them on the label.

At present there is virtually no way in which a parent can learn from the label what the complete contents of a package may be. The solution to this problem is obviously to require full disclosure of ingredients on the package label, however even with mounting public concern, it will be a long time, if ever, before full disclosure is a reality.

There are several things which the parents of an allergic child should consider when buying packaged foods:

the labeled contents of the package
chemicals used in processing the food
packaging materials
chemicals leached into the food from the packaging materials.

The FDA allows some leaching (transfer) of chemicals from the packaging materials into the food. Listed below are substances which can migrate into food.

Substances migrating from cotton and cotton fabrics used in dry food packaging:

acetic acid	beef tallow
calcium chloride	coconut oil, refined
corn dextrin	cornstarch
fish oil (hydrogenated)	gelatin
Japan wax	lard
lard oil	lecithin
peanut oil	potato starch
stearic acid	talc
tallow(hydrogenated)	wheat starch

Substances migrating to food from paper and paperboard products:

acetic acid	casein
clay (kaolin)	cornstarch
corn syrup	dextrin
glycerin	invert sugar
sorbitol	soy protein (isolated)
starch, acid modified	starch, pregelatinized
starch, unmodified	talc

Some changes have taken place in the last few years which are to the consumer's advantage. Ice cream which is sold interstate must now carry a more complete list of ingredients in descending order of predominance, as must many other packaged goods. (Before this, more than 30 additives to ice cream were allowed to be used without mention.)

There are still close to 300 products that, since made from "standard" recipes, enjoy the privilege of not having to list all their necessary and optional ingredients on the label. Many substances still remain invisible under the label of "artificial and natural colors and flavors." (See tables.)

INTRODUCTION TO TABLES OF ADDITIVES

There are literally thousands of food additives used in the foods we eat today. According to the FDA Codes, some substances are considered additives in one food and not another; there are also additives which must be labeled in one food and not in another; there are intentional additives and unintentional additives. The qualifications are seemingly endless.

What is an additive?

The *CRC Handbook of Food Additives* states that a food additive "is a substance or mixture of substances, other than a basic foodstuff, which is present in food as a result of any aspect of production, processing, storage or packing. The term does not include chance contaminants."[1]

Food additives have been used for centuries. Salting meats and the addition of large amounts of sugar to fruit in preserves and jams were methods of preserving food used early in history. The use of spices even influenced the course of that history.

The additives used currently have many functions. The *Federal Code of Regulations*, Title 21, classifies additives according to their function as preservatives, coloring and flavoring agents, antimicrobial agents, antioxidants, emulsifiers, sequestrants, stabilizers, anticaking agents, sweeteners, bleaches, drying agents, humectants, pH control agents, texturizers and so on.

The following tables should give you an idea of what the various additives are, and where they can be found in food.

A complete list of synthetic flavors may be found in the *CRC Handbook of Food Additives* published by the Chemical Rubber Company, 1980. As a closing note to this section, I am including an excerpt from the *Federal Code of Regulations*, Title 21, Food and Drugs:

Section 101.6 Label designation of ingredients for standardized foods.

(a) There is significant consumer interest that labels of standardized foods bear complete information on the ingredients contained in the food. In the absence of legal authority to require that

209

the label bear such information, the Food and Drug Administration encourages all manufacturers, packers, and distributors to voluntarily make such disclosure.

(b) The Food and Drug Administration intends to amend the definitions and standards of identity of food by setting into motion as rapidly as possible the provisions of Section 401 of the Act to require label declaration of all optional ingredients with the exception of optional spices, flavorings, and colorings which may continue to be designated as such without specific ingredient declaration.

(c) Statutory authority does not exist to require the declaration of mandatory ingredients on the label of standardized foods.[2]

[1]Food Protection Committee, 1959, *Principles and Procedures for Evaluating the Safety of Food Additives,* NAS NRC Publication #750.

[2]21 U.S.C.R., Ch. 1: Food and Drug Administration, Sec. 101.6, 1979.

Type	Definition	Additive	Found In
Antimicrobial agent	inhibits growth of microbes which would contaminate the food	Benzoic acid	beverages, purees, concentrates
		ATP	margarine, salad dressings, mayonnaise
		sodium benzoate	margarine, pie filling, dressings
		sorbates	beverages, dairy prod., baked goods, fruits
		ethyl and propyl paraben	beverages, syrups purees, baked goods
		sulfites	beverages, dried fruits and veg., pickles
		acetates, diacetates	baked goods, salad dressings, relishes
		nitrite, nitrate	processed meat and fish
Antioxidants	prevents breakdown of ingredients due to oxidation	BHA	beverages, mixes, cereals, potato flakes
		BHT	enriched rice, chewing gum base, processed food
		propyl gallate THBP (trihydrox-butyropgenone) DLTDP (dilauryl thiodipropionate)	oil, meat prod., dried potatoes, chew. gum
		gum guaiac	oil-containing foods
		tocopherals	oils
		lecithin	baked goods, ice cream, margarine, chocolate
PH control agent	changes or maintains acidity or basicity of food	acetic acid	vinegars
		adipic acid	bottled beverages, gelatin desserts, oils
		lactic acid	olives, cheese, fruit beverages, frozen desserts, powdered & condensed milk
		sorbic acid	soft drinks, syrup, jelly, cake, margarine, frosting
		fumaric acid	soft drink mixes, dry gelatin, pudding and pie fillings, candy, leavening agents

Type	Definition	Additive	Found In
Sequestrants	combines with poly-valent metal ions to improve stability and quality of food product	acetic acid adipic acid	
		albumin benzoic acid	sandwich spreads, processed fruits and vegetables, fruit juices, canned shellfish
		casein	
		EDTA	beer, soft drinks
		glutamic acid glycine	artificially sweetened soft drinks
		sodium citrate	gelatin dessert, jam, candy, ice cream
		sodium phosphate	imitation sausage
Gums	material that can be dissolved or dispersed in water to give viscosity to solutions	gum arabic (acacia)	candy, powdered drink mixes, beer, ice cream
		karaya gum	whipped products, sausage, ice cream
		larch and ghatti	salad dressings, syrups with butter
		tragacanth	acidic foods (salad dressings)
	seaweed	agar	icings, baked goods, whipped cream, ice cream
		algin	candy, ice cream, cheese, yogurt, whipped cream
		carageenan	instant breakfast, formulas, sour cream, ice cream
		furcellaran	puddings and desserts
	seed or root	guar	beverages, dough, ice cream, whipped topping
		locust bean	doughs and mixes, salad dressings, ice cream
		psyllium seed quince seed	
	misc.	pectin	jellies, canned frosting, yogurt
		gelatin	beverages, gelatin desserts, yogurt, ice cream
		starch	baby foods, pie fillings, icings, dessert mixes
		xanthan gum	breads

Type	Definition	Additive	Found In
Colors	used to enhance or give color to, or to preserve the color of food or drugs	Erythrosine (Red #3)	candy, baked goods, cherries in acid solutions
		Ponceau Sx (Red #4)	maraschino cherries (also drugs)
		Red #40 (Allura Red AC)	candy, gelatin, baked goods, soda
		Brilliant blue FCF (#1)	baked goods, beverages, candy
		Indigotine (Blue #2)	beverages, candy
		Tartrazine (Yellow #5)	baked goods, candy, gelatin desserts, drugs
		Sunset Yellow FCF (#6)	baked goods, candy, gelatin, beverages, sausage
		Fast Green FCF (#3)	
		Orange B	frankfurters (casing)
		Citrus Red #2	orange skins
		ferrous gluconate	olives
		beta carotene	butter, nondairy creamers, margarine, shortening
		algae meal	eggs and chicken (as feed to enhance yellow)
		annato extract (tree)	cheese, ice cream
		caramel* cottonseed flour fruit and vegetable juice	ubiquitous
		grape skin extract	beverages
		paprika (from pepper)	frankfurters
		saffron (from poppy)	rice, baked goods
		titanium dioxide	to whiten, in snack crackers, sugar syrup
		turmeric carrot oil	rice products
		carbon black beet powder	bakery products
Flavors (see table for natural flavors)			

*Caramel can be made from any of the following: dextrose, lactose, malt syrup, molasses, starch, sucrose.

213

MEDICATIONS

The days are gone when the physician both diagnosed illnesses and made up his own medicines. In the twentieth century, the physician makes a diagnosis and decides on a treatment, but the medication is provided by any of the many pharmaceutical companies. While medications must be tested for efficacy and side-effects (by law), the companies cannot be familiar with every child's particular sensitivities.

Both allergic and non-allergic children can react to medication, however parents of allergic children have a specific problem which has not yet been addressed by either the FDA or many pharmaceutical companies.

When a child has an allergic reaction to a prescription or non-prescription drug, it can be devastating. The question should then be asked whether the drug itself caused the reaction, or whether it was one of the "excipients" (inactive ingredients) in the medication. As this information is not listed in the physician's references, many simply change the prescription to another medication and the quest for an acceptable treatment is continued.

If the physician and parents knew the ingredients of the medications, both the initial and possible subsequent reactions could be more easily avoided. This is rarely the case however. While the pharmaceutical companies are usually willing to answer specific questions from health professionals, many do not maintain 24-hour availability. Other companies consider the excipients used in their products to be "proprietary and confidential information" and will not disclose the ingredients to the public. Most will, however, answer physicians' questions if requested. A few companies will disclose this information to parents on an individual basis and maintain a consumer information service. Some pharmaceutical houses do not know the excipients in their products since they purchase them and only demand that all ingredients be of FDA approved quality.

What are these excipients and why are they important?

Medicines are often available in different forms, using alternate methods of delivery (i.e. tablet vs. liquid). The reasons for using the different forms are many. Sometimes a medication must be released at a particular site in the digestive system to be most

214

effective. Excipients assure that this will happen. They also regulate the length of time the medication remains in the bloodstream and the rate of absorption by the body. Many medications are coated to protect the mouth from irritating substances, to avoid unpleasant tastes, to assure control over the rate of disintegration, or to protect the medication itself. Each of these should be considered when dealing with a child with extreme sensitivities.

Many substances may be added to the active ingredient in the medication. These excipients act as:

Binders—blended with tablet ingredients to hold them together, allowing the tablet to disintegrate at the proper time.

Buffers—maintaining a desired pH (level of acidity or alkalinity).

Colors and flavors—aiding in patient acceptance and identification of medication.

Preservatives—preventing deterioration or oxidation of the medicine.

Disintegrators—causing the vehicle to break apart and release the active ingredient into the digestive tract at the correct time.

Emulsifying agents and suspending agents—allowing miniscule particles of undissolved medication to be suspended in a liquid vehicle.

When I began working on this section of the book, I assumed (rather naively) that the pharmaceutical companies would be willing to assist, simply because of the possibility of avoiding adverse reactions to their products. While most companies were quite helpful, some provided me with interesting reasons for not cooperating. As one company spokesperson said, "There is considerable disagreement. . . as to the wisdom of providing information to patients which could well cause them undue alarm and might possibly interfere with the physician-patient relationship." And another company replied that, ". . .when considering the inevitable product formulation changes, additions and deletions, it may be somewhat difficult to maintain current records of all the hundreds of products we market as related to numerous excipients." One company even replied that they do not ask their suppliers the origin of the materials they use, but simply require that these materials comply with federal regulations.

A more reasonable explanation for refusing to divulge the ingredients of their products came from a spokesman from one pharmaceutical house, "Again, our concern is that any published list, particularly in a book, may be misleading. Either the presence or absence of a product can be equally misleading and potentially dangerous to a highly allergic individual. Ingredients in our products do change at a higher frequency than is generally recognized by the public. Over the course of the last several years, cyclamates, saccharin, numerous dyes (FD&C Red #2, FD&C Yellow #5, etc.) chloroform, flavors, preservatives, anti-oxidents, certain coated vitamins, have been removed from some of our products. In some instances this was necessitated by FDA action (i.e. saccharin), reported allergies (FD&C Yellow #5), competitive reasons or unavailability of these ingredients from our vendors." Abbott provides a toll-free number for "health care professionals" to call for information on the allergic potential of their products.

When I later requested an updated list from another major pharmaceutical company, they replied that ". . . the information which you received is still valid and would be true today. Please understand that any changes in formulation must be cleared by the FDA and any change in a formula would create a new product."

In the interim between my first inquiries and the final updates, very few changes in product formulation were indicated by the companies who responded to the queries. However, it should be noted that this section is intended only as a guide to inform the parent of the various components which may be present in medication and make him/her aware of the potential problems.

It is absolutely necessary to contact the pharmaceutical company for exact information pertaining to any medication.

Ultimately it is your child who will be affected by the medication taken. Know what it is your child is swallowing. Have the physician check with the company, and ask the pharmacist to supply you with the lot number of the prescribed medication so you will be able to give specific information to the company should you need to consult them.

INTRODUCTION TO THE TABLES

This section of the book has been divided into three parts. The first is comprised of tables of products. Medications produced by each company are listed together.

The second group of listings contain those medications (again by company) for which the manufacturer supplied information about only a few excipients.

The last section contains only the manufacturer's name, a product listing and (if available) an emergency telephone number. These companies felt that the excipient content of medications is "proprietary and confidential" information and were unwilling that it be distributed. Some will answer patient queries, and others will only respond to requests from "qualified health personnel."

PRODUCT INFORMATION

E.R. SQUIBB & SONS, INC.

Over the Counter Products that Contain No Sugar
Aspirin tablets
Brewer's yeast tablets
Castor oil
Cod liver oil
Mint-flavored cod liver oil
Cod liver oil capsules
Golden Bounty
All insulin formulations
Milk of Magnesia
Mint-O-Mag
Mineral oil
Niacin 500 mg.
Pronestyl capsules 500 mg.
Pronestyl tablets
Rau-Sed tablets
Rezipas
Saccharin tablets

Sumycin capsules (L)
Sumycin tablets
Suppositories, glycerin
Sweeta liquid
Sweeta tablets
Teslac tablets (L)
Trigesic tablets
Valadol tablets (L)
Veetids 250 tablets (L)
Veetids 500 tablets (L)
Velosef 250 capsules (L)
Velosef 500 capsules (L)
Vesprin High Potency Suspension
Vesprin tablets(L)
Vigran capsules
Vitamin A capsules
Vitamin B_1 tablets USP (L)
Vitamin B_{12} capsules
Vitamin C orange-flavored tablets (Tablets do contain sugar.)
Vitamin C tablets (Ascorbic Acid tablets, USP)
Vitamin E capsules
Wheat germ oil capsules

(L) - Products which contain lactose

E.R. SQUIBB & SONS, INC.

Oral Liquid Formulations that contain No Alcohol
Castor oil
Cod liver oil
Mint-flavored cod liver oil
Gastrografin
Kenacort diacetate syrup
Milk of Magnesia
Mint-O-Mag
Mineral oil
Mysteclin-F syrup
Noctec syrup
Pentids for syrup

Pentids 400 for syrup
Principen 125 for oral suspension
Principen 250 for oral suspension
Sumycin syrup
Terfonyl suspension
Theragran liquid
Veetids 125 for oral solution
Veetids 250 for oral solution
Velosef 125 for oral susupension
Velosef 250 for oral suspension
Vesprin High Potency Suspension

E.R. SQUIBB & SONS, INC.

Formulations that do Not Contain Sucrose or Dextrose
Aspirin tablets
B complex with C capsules (L)
Brewer's yeast tablets
Castor oil
Cod liver oil
Cod liver oil capsules
Mint-flavored cod liver oil
Diagnex Blue (Caffeine and Sodium Benzoate Tablets (L))
Ethril 250 mg. tablets
Ethril 500 mg. tablets
Florinef acetate tablets (L)
Gastrograrin
Golden Bounty vitamins
Hydrea capsules (L)
Kenacort tablets (L)
Kenalog in Orabase
Milk of Magnesia
Mint-O-Mag
Mineral oil
Mycostatin oral tablets
Mycostatin vaginal tablets (L)
Mysteclin F capsules (L)
Naturetin tablets (L)
Neomycin sulfate tablets (L)
Niacin tablets (L)

219

Noctec capsules
Nydrazid tablets (L)
Oragratin sodium capsules
Ora-Testryl tablets (L)
Pentids tablets (L)
Pentids 400 tablets (L)
Pentids 800 tablets
Principen 250 capsules (L)
Principen 500 capsules (L)
Principen with Probenecid capsules
Pronestyl capsules 250 mg. (L)
Vitamin A capsules
Vitamin E capsules
Wheat germ capsules

(L) – Products which contain lactose

ROCHE LABORATORIES

Free of Corn Starch or Other Derivatives of Corn
Accutane™ (isotretinoin/Roche) – containing hydrogenated
   vegetable oil
Alurate Elixer (aprobarbital/Roche)
Arfonad ™ Ampuls (trimethophan camsylate/Roche)
Bactrim™ I.V. Infusion(trimethoprim and sulfamethoxazole/
   Roche)
Bactrim™ Pediatric suspension(trimethoprim and sulfam
ethoxazole/ Roche)
Bactrim™ Suspension (40 mg. trimethoprim and 200 mg.
   sulfamethoxazole/Roche)
Berocca™ –C Ampuls
Berocca™–C Vials
Berocca™ –C 500
Berocca™ –C Plus Injection
Berocca™ Parenteral Nutrition
Berocca™ Plus tablets
Berocca™ Tablets
Berocca™ –WS
Clonopin™ Tablets (clonazepam/Roche) – all strengths

Efudex™ Cream 5% (flouracil/Roche)
Efudex™ Solution 2% (flouracil/Roche)
Efudex ™ Solution 5% (flouracil/Roche)
Emeyt ™ (estramustine phosphate sodium/Roche)
Flourouracil Ampuls (5-flourouracil/Roche)
FUDR(floxuridine/Roche)
Gantanol™ Suspension (sulfamethoxazole/Roche)
Gantrisin™ Ampuls 5 ml. (sulfisoxazole diolamine/Roche)
Gantrisin™ Ampuls 10 ml. (sulfisoxazole diolamine/Roche)
Gantrisin™ Ophthalmic ointment 4%(sulfisoxazole diolam
ine/ Roche)
Gantrisin™ Ophthalmic solution 4% (sulfisoxazole diolamine/
Roche)
Gantrisin™ Pediatric suspension (acetyl sulfisoxazole/Roche)
Gantrisin™ Syrup (acetyl sulfisoxazole/Roche)
Larobec™ Tablets
Larodopa™ Tablets (levodopa/Roche) – all strengths
Levo-Dromoran™ Ampuls (levorphanol tartrate/Roche) CII
Levo-Dromoran™ Vials (levomphanol tartrate/Roche) CII
Librium™ Injectable (chlordiazepoxide HCl/Roche) CIV
Limbitrol ™ Tablets, 25 mg. (chlordiazepoxide and amitrip-
tyline HCl/Roche)
Lipo Gantrisin™ Suspension (acetyl sulfisoxazole/Roche)
Lorfan™ Injectable Ampuls (levallorphan tartrate/Roche)
Lorfan™ Injectable Vials (levallorphan tartrate/Roche)
Mestinon™ Injectable Ampuls(pyridostigmine bromide/
Roche)
Mestinon™ Syrup (pyridostigmine bromide/Roche)
Mestinon™ Tablets 60 mg. (pyridostigmine bromide/Roche)
Mestinon™ Timespan Tablets, 180 mg. (pyridostigmine
bromide/Roche)
Nipride™ Injectable Vials (sodium nitroprusside/Roche)
Nisentil™ Ampuls (alphaprodine hydrochloride/Roche) – all
strengths CII
Nisentil™ Vials (alphaprodine hydrochloride/Roche) – all
strengths CII
Pantopon™ Injectable Ampuls (hydrochlorides of opium
alkaloids/Roche) CII
Prostigmin™ Ampuls (neostigmine bromide/Roche) – all
strengths

Ronakion™ Ampuls (phytonadione/Roche) – all strengths
Roniacol™ Elixer (nicotinyl alcohol/Roche)
Roniacol™ Timespan Tablets, 150 mg. (nicotinyl alcohol tartrate/Roche)
Solatene™ Capsules (beta-carotene/Roche)
Synkayvite™ Injectable Ampuls (menadiol sodium diphosphate/Roche)–all strengths
Taractan™ Concentrate (chlorprothixene/Roche)
Taractan™ Parenteral Ampuls (chlorprothixene/Roche)
Tensilon™ Ampuls(edrophonium chloride/Roche)all strengths
Valium™ Injectable Ampuls (diazepam/Roche) CIV
Valium™ Injectable Tel-E-Ject Disposable Syringes (diazepam/Roche) CIV
Valium™ Injectable Vials (diazepam/Roche) CIV
Valrelease™ (diazepam/Roche) CIV
Vi-Penta™ Infant Drops
Vi-Penta™ F Infant Drops
Vi-Penta™ Multivitamin Drops
Vi-Penta™ F Multivitamin Drops
Vi-Penta™ F Chewable Tablets

SANDOZ PHARMACEUTICAL DIVISION PRODUCTS

Product contains	Milk	Corn	Pork
Asborn G Inlay Tabs		starch	
Belladenal Tablet	lactose	starch	gelatin
Belladenal-S Tablets	lactose	starch	gelatin
Bellafoline Ampuls	lactose		
Bellafoline Tablets	lactose		
Bellergal Tablets	lactose	starch	gelatin
Bellergal-S Tablets	lactose		
Cafergot Tablets	lactose	starch	
Cafergot PB Tablets		starch	
Cafergot PB Suppositories	lactose		
Fiogesic Tablets	lactose	starch	
Fiorinal Capsules		starch	gelatin capsule
Fiorinal Codeine Capsules		starch	gelatin capsule

222

Fiorinal Tablets	lactose		
Gris-PEG Tablets 125 mg	lactose		
Gynergen Tablets	lactose	starch	
Hydergine Sublingual Tablets		starch	gelatin
Hydergine Oral Tablets	lactose	starch	
Mellaril Tablets 10, 15, 25, 50, 200 mg	lactose	starch	gelatin
Mellaril Tablets 100 & 150 mg.	lactose	starch	
Mesantoin Tablets	lactose	starch	gelatin
Metaprel Tablets	lactose	starch	
Methergine Tablets	lactose	starch	
Pamelor Capsules		starch	gelatin capsule
Parlodel Capsules		starch	gelatin capsule
Parlodel Tablets	lactose	starch	
Restoril Capsules	lactose		gelatin capsule
Sanorex Tablets	lactose	starch	
Sansert Tablets	lactose	starch	gelatin
Tavist-1 Tablets	lactose	starch	
Tavist Tablets	lactose	starch	
Tavist-D Tablets	lactose	starch	
Trest Tablets	lactose	starch	
Visken Tablets		starch	

SANDOZ PHARMACEUTICALS DIVISION PRODUCTS WITHOUT INGREDIENTS FROM EGGS, WHEAT, CORN, MILK, PORK OR PEANUTS

Asbron G Elixir
Bellafoline Ampuls
Bellafoline Tablets
Cafergot Suppositories
Cedilanid-D Injection
D.H.E. 45 Injection
Diapid Nasal Spray
Gris-PEG Tablets 250 mg.
Gynergen Injection
Hydergine Liquid

Klorvess Effervescent Granules
Klorvess Effervescent Tablets
Klorvess 108 Liquid
Mellaril Concentrate
Mellaril Suspension
Metaprel Syrup
Metaprel Metered Dose Inhaler
Metaprel Inhalant Solution 5%
Methergine Injection
Neo-Calglucon Syrup
Pamelor Solution
Syntocinon Injection
Syntocinon Nasal Spray

McNEIL CONSUMER PRODUCTS COMPANY

Products Containing Corn Starch
Regular strength TYLENOL tablets and capsules
Extra-strength TYLENOL tablets and capsules
SINE-AID tablets
CoTYLENOL tablets and capsules

Products Containing Animal Products (Calcium or Magnesium Stearate)
Regular strength TYLENOL tablets and capsules
Extra-strength TYLENOL tablets and capsules
SINE-AID tablets
CoTYLENOL tablets and capsules
Chewable TYLENOL tablets

Products Containing Citric Acid
Extra-strength adult TYLENOL liquid
CoTYLENOL liquid
Children's TYLENOL elixir
Chewable TYLENOL tablets
TYLENOL drops
Children's CoTYLENOL liquid

No Products Contain Milk or Milk Derivatives.
No Products Contain Other Grain or Grain Derivatives.

USV PHARMACEUTICAL COMPANY

Products Containing Lactose
Arlidin™ (nylidrin HCl) 6 mg. and 12 mg. tablets
Cerespan™ (papaverine HCl) 150 capsules
C.V.P. and duo C.V.P. capsules (brands of bioflavonoids, 100
  mg. and 200 mg. respectively)
Demi-Regroton™ (chlorthalidone/reserpine) 25 mg. chlorthal-
  idone; 0.1125 mg. reserpine; tablet
Hygroton™ (chlorthalidone USP) 25 mg., 50 mg. and 100 mg.
  tablets
Nitrospan™ (nitroglycerin) 2.5 mg. and 6.5 mg. capsules
Pertofrane™ (desipramine hydrochloride NF) 25 mg. and 50
  mg. capsules
Presamine™ (imipramine hydrochloride USP) 25 mg. and 50
  mg. tablets
Regroton™ (chlorthalidone/reserpine) 50 mg. chlorthalidone;
  0.25 mg. reserpine; tablet

Products Containing Corn Starch
Arlidin™ (nylidrin HCl) 6 mg. and 12 mg. tablets
Azolid™ (phenylbutazone USP) 100 mg. tablets and capsules
Cerespan™ (papaverine HCl) 150 capsules
C.V.P. capsules
Duo C.V.P. capsules
Doriden™ (glutethimide USP) (0.5 g. capsules)
Histaspan™ Plus capsules
Histapan-D™ capsules
Hygroton™ (chlorthalidone USP) 25 mg., 50 mg. and 100 mg.
  tablets
Nitrospan™ (nitroglycerin) 2.5 mg. and 6.5 mg. capsules
Oxalid™ (pxyphenbutazone) 100 mg. tablets
Presamine™ (imipramine hydrochloride USP) 25 mg. and 50
  mg. tablets
Regroton™ (chlorathalidone USP 50 mg./reserpine USP 0.25
  mg.) tablets
Demi-Regroton™ (chlorathalidone USP 25 mg./reserpine
  USP 0.125 mg.) tablets
Thyrolar™ (liotrix, Armour) 1/4, 1/2, 1, 2, and 3 tablets

225

Products Not Containing Dyes

Acthar™ Lyophilized 25 and 40 IU (Corticotropin for Injection)

H.P. Acthar™ Gel 20, 40, and 80 IU/ML (Repository Corticotropin Injection)

Albuminar™– 5 (Normal Serum Albumin [human] USP 5%)

Albuminar™– 20 (Normal Serum Albumin [human] USP 20%)

Albuminar™– 25 (Normal Serum Albumin [human] USP 25%)

Aquasol™ A Parenteral (water-miscible Vitamin A)

Aquasol™ A Drops (Vitamin A in aqueous solution)

Arlidin™ (Nylidrin HCl)

Arm-A-Med™ /Arm-A-Vial™ (Respiratory Therapy System)

Armour™ Thyroid (Throid, USP) tablets

Barotrast™ (Barium Sulfate, USP)

Biozyme-C™ (Collagenase Enzyme)

Calcimar™ (Calcitonin Salmon)

Chrometrace™ (Chromic Chloride Injection, USP)

Clysodrast™ (Bisacodyl and Tannnic Acid)

Coppertrace™ (Cupric Chloride Injection, USP)

DDAVP™ (Desmopressin Acetate)

Demi-Regroton™ (Chlorthalidone 50 mg., Reserpine 0.25 mg.)

Dialume™ capsules (Aluminum Hydroxide Powder)

Doriden™ (Glutethimide, USP) tablets (0.25 & 0.5 g.)

Esophotrast™ (Barium Sulfate)

Factorate™ (Antihemophilic Factor [human] USP dried)

Factorate™ Generation II (Antihemophilic Factor [human] USP dried)

Gammar™ (Immune Serum Globulin [human] USP)

Gamulin™ Rh (Rh D Immune Globulin [human])

Hygroton™ (Chlorthalidone, USP) 100 mg.

Levothroid™ (Levothyroxine sodium, USP) tablets (0.05 mg.)

Levothroid™ injectable (Levothyroxine sodium, USP)

Mangatrace™ (Manganese Chloride Injection, USP)

Mini-Gamulin™ Rh (Rh D Immune Globulin [human])

Oratrast™ (Barium Sulfate)

Oxalid™ (oxyphenbutazone USP) tablets (100 mg.)

Plasma-Plex™ (Plasma Protein Fraction [human] USP)

Thrombinar™ (Bovine thrombin)

Thyrar™ (Thyroid Equivalent to USP Powder) tablets (1/2 & 2 grain)

Thytropar™ (Thyrotropin for injection)
Zinctrace™ (Zinc Chloride Injection, USP)

Vitamins

At present, not all companies routinely publish complete lists of product information (list includes source, excipients, sweeteners, and coatings). Those who do are :

WILLIAM T. THOMPSON COMPANY
P.O. Box 6201
Carson, CA 90749

Among their products are tapioca-base, corn-free Vitamin C tablets.

NUTRI-COLOGY
2336 C Stanwell Circle
Concord, CA 94520

Nutri-Cology also produces hypoallergenic (labeled) vitamin supplements which contain no binders or excipients. (Pull-apart capsules are used.)

SCHIFF BIO FOOD PRODUCTS, MFG.
Moonachie, NJ 07074

Among their products are rice-based B vitamins and folic acid tablets, and Vitamin C from rose hips (no starch, sugar, or preservatives).

Product	Corn	Beef or Pork	Milk
Albion Chelated Calcium tablets		stearic acid	
Albion Chelated Iron Plex tablets	ascorbic acid	stearic acid	
Albion Chelated Iron tablets		stearic acid	
Albion Chelated Magnesium tablets		stearic acid	
Albion Chelated Manganese tablets & capsules		gelatin, stearic acid	
Albion Chelated Multi-Vita-Min capsules	ascorbic acid	gelatin, stearic acid	
Albion Chelated MultiMin tablets		stearic acid	
Albion Chelated Potassium tablets		stearic acid	
Albion Chelated Tri-Mins tablets		stearic acid	
Albion Chelated Zinc tabs & caps		gelatin, stearic acid	
Boehringer Ingleheim Alupent syrup			
Boehringer Ingleheim Catapres tablets	starch	gelatin, glycerine	lactose
Boehringer Ingleheim Dulcolax tablets	starch	gelatin, stearates, glycerine	lactose
Bristol Naldecon CX		unspecified	
Bristol Naldecon drops			
Bristol Naldecon DX		unspecified	
Bristol Naldecon EX			
Bristol Naldecon pediatric syrup			
Bristol Naldecon syrup			
Bristol Naldecon tablets	unspecified	gelatin	unspecified
Bristol Naldegesic	unspecified	unspecified	
Bristol Naldetuss			
Bristol Polycillin caps			unspecified
Bristol Polycillin suspension			
Bristol Polymox caps			unspecified
Bristol Polymox suspension			
E.I. du Pont de Nemours Coumadin tabs, 10.0 mg	starch	stearates	pregelatinized lactose

Wheat or Grains	Dyes	Gums and Resins	Miscellaneous
alcohol			
	FD&C red #40	methyl paraben, propyl paraben, hydroxyethyl cellulose hydroxyethyl	sodium metabisulfite, saccharin, sorbitol
	FD&C yellow #6	methylparaben, propylparaben	
sucrose	FD&C yellow #5, FD&C yellow #6 lake, titanium dioxide	carnauba wax, acacia, shellac, white wax, cellulose acetate	talc
	unspecified		
	unspecified		
	unspecified		
	unspecified		
	unspecified		
	unspecified		
	unspecified		
	unspecified		
	unspecified (shell only)		
	unspecified		
	unspecified (shell only)		
	unspecified		
			tapioca

Product	Corn	Beef or Pork	Milk
E.I. du Pont de Nemours Coumadin tabs, 2.0 mg	starch	stearates	pregelatinized lactose
E.I. du Pont de Nemours Coumadin tabs, 2.5 mg	starch	stearates	pregelatinized lactose
E.I. du Pont de Nemours Coumadin tabs, 5.0 mg	starch	stearates	pregelatinized lactose
E.I. du Pont de Nemours Coumadin tabs, 7.5 mg	starch	stearates	pregelatinized lactose
E.I. du Pont de Nemours Endecon tabs	starch	stearates	pregelatinized lactose
E.I. du Pont de Nemours Endotussin-NN Ped. syrup		glycerine	
E.I. du Pont de Nemours Endotussin-NN syrup		glycerine	
E.I. du Pont de Nemours Hycomine Ped. syrup		glycerine	
E.I. du Pont de Nemours Hycomine syrup		glycerine	
E.I. du Pont de Nemours Hycomine tablets	starch	stearates	
E.I. du Pont de Nemours Hycotuss Expectorant		glycerine	
E.I. du Pont de Nemours Percodan tabs	starch		
Eli Lilly & Co. Enseals	starch	gelatin, stearates, stearic acid	
Eli Lilly & Co. Histadyl E.C.		glycerine	
Eli Lilly & Co. Ilosone chewable 125 mg		stearates, stearic acid	
Eli Lilly & Co. Ilosone chewable 250 mg		stearates, stearic acid	

Wheat or Grains	Dyes	Gums and Resins	Miscellaneous
starch	FD&C blue lake #2, FD&C red lake #40		
starch	FD&C yellow #6		
starch	FD&C red #3 lake, FD&C yellow #6 lake		
starch	FD&C yellow #6 lake, FD&C yellow #10 lake		
	FD&C yellow #10, FD&C blue #2		
alcohol, sugar	FD&C red #40		sorbitol
alcohol, sugar	FD&C red #40, FD&C yellow #6, FD&C blue #2		sorbitol, art. cherry
	FD&C green #3, FD&C yellow #10		sorbitol, sod. saccharin
	FD&C yellow #6, FD&C red #40		sorbitol, sod. saccharin
	FD&C red #40, FD&C red #40 lake		cherry, dry
alcohol, liquid sugar	FD&C yellow #6, FD&C red #40		sorbitol, soc. saccharin, art. butterscotch
	FD&C yellow #6 lake, FD&C yellow #10 lake		
	FD&C red #7, FD&C yellow #5	methylcellulose, acacia, acetylated monoglycerides, cellulose, polyethelyne	sucrose, talc, castor oil, white wax
alcohol	FD&C red #33, FD&C yellow #6		marasc. cherry, caramel, vanillin, sucrose, saccharin
	FD&C red #40, FD&C yellow #6, FD&C yellow #5	microcrystalline cellulose	sucrose, lemon fl. #5, imit. cinnamon, imit. marasc. cherry, peppermint, mannitol, citric acid
	FD&C yellow #5, FD&C yellow #6, FD&C red #40	microcrystalline cellulose	sucrose, lemon #5, imit. cinnamon, imit. marasc. cherry, peppermint, mannitol, citric acid

Product	Corn	Beef or Pork	Milk
Eli Lilly & Co. Ilosone for oral susp. 125 mg per 5 ml			
Eli Lilly & Co. Ilosone liquid 125 mg per 5 ml			
Eli Lilly & Co. Ilosone liquid 250 mg per 5 ml			
Eli Lilly & Co. Ilosone Pulvules 125 mg		gelatin, stearates	
Eli Lilly & Co. Ilosone Pulvules 250 mg		gelatin, stearates	
Eli Lilly & Co. Ilosone Ready-Mixed drops 100 mg per 5 ml			
Eli Lilly & Co. Ilosone tabs, 500 mg	starch	stearates, glycerine	
Fleming Congress Jr. T.D. caps		gelatin	
Fluritab Corp. Fluoritab Liquid			
Fluritab Corp. Fluoritab tabs			lactose
Glaxo Inc. Theobid Duracap			
Glaxo Inc. Amesec caps	starch		
Glaxo Inc. Vi-Zinc			
Glaxo Inc. Vicon-C, Vicon-Plus, Vicon Forte			
Hoyt Laboratories Luride Lozi-tabs		stearates (pork)	
Hoyt Laboratories Luride-SF Lozi-tabs		stearates (pork)	
Hoyt Laboratories Phos-Flur Rinse, Cherry, Orange, Lime			
Hoyt Laboratories Phos-Flur Rinse, Cinnamon			

Wheat or Grains	Dyes	Gums and Resins	Miscellaneous
	FD&C yellow #6, FD&C red #3		sucrose, lemon #5, imit. cinnamon, imit. marasc. cherry, peppermint, citric acid
	FD&C yellow #6	methylparaben, butylparaben, propylparaben, cellulose	sucrose, orange oil valencia
	FD&C red #40	methylparaben, butylparaben, propylparaben, cellulose	imit. guarana, imit. cherry, imit. cherry pit, sucrose, citric acid, sodium saccharin
	FD&C red #3, FD&C yellow #5, FD&C yellow #6, titanium dioxide	silica gel	talc
	FD&C red #3, FD&C yellow #5, FD&C yellow #6, titanium dioxide	silica gel	talc
	FD&C yellow #6	methylparaben, propylparaben, cellulose	sucrose, orange oil valencia, citric acid
	FD&C red #3 lake, FD&C yellow #5 lake, FD&C red #30 lake, titanium dioxide	hydroxypropyl-methylcellulose, hydroxypropyl-cellulose	
sucrose	FD&C yellow	shellac	
			multi-fruit flavoring
insoluble sucrose	FD&C blue #1		
starch			silicon
	unspecified		talc
			talc
	unspecified		mannitol, sorbitol, unspecified flavoring agents
			mannitol, sorbitol
	unspecified		sorbitol, unspecified flavoring agents
	unspecified		unspecified flavoring agents

233

Product	Corn	Beef or Pork	Milk
Hoyt Laboratories Thera-Flur Gel Drops			
Hoyt Laboratories Thera-Flur-N Gel Drops			
Laser Inc. Dallergy caps		gelatin, stearates	
Laser Inc. Dallergy syrup		glycerine	
Laser Inc. Donatussin DC syrup			
Laser Inc. Donatussin drops			
Laser Inc. Donatussin syrup			
Laser Inc. Fumatinic caps	starch	gelatin	
Laser Inc. Fumerin tabs		gelatin, stearates	
Laser Inc. KIE syrup			
Laser Inc. Myobid caps		gelatin	
Laser Inc. Respaire-SR caps	starch	gelatin	
Laser Inc. Theospan SR caps	starch	gelatin	
Laser Inc. Theostat SO syrup			
Laser Inc. Theostat tabs		gelatin, stearates	
Laser Inc., Dallergy tabs		stearates	
Marion Labs Cardizem tablets 60 mg	starch		lactose
Marion Labs Duotrate caps	starch		

Wheat or Grains	Dyes	Gums and Resins	Miscellaneous
	unspecified		sorbitol, unspecified flavoring agents
			sorbitol
	FD&C red #3, titanium dioxide	pharmaceutical glaze, carboxy methylcellulose	cane sugar, mannitol, citric acid
	FD&C blue #1, FD&C red #33	propylene glycol	imit. grape flavor, cane sugar, citric acid
	FD&C red #40	propylene glycol	cane sugar, menthol, vanillin, art. apricot, art. pineapple, cocillana fluid ext. citric acid
	FD&C yellow #6	propylene glycol, propyl paraben	cane sugar, imit. fruit, custard, saccharin
	FD&C red #33	propylene glycol, propyl paraben	cane sugar, wild cherry, vanilla, citrus, saccharin
	titanium dioxide, FD&C red #3, FD&C yellow #6		cane sugar
	titanium dioxide, FD&C red #3, FD&C blue #1	beeswax Lac resin, carnauba wax	cane sugar, potato starch
	FD&C blue #1, FD&C yellow #10		cherry fl., citric acid, sorbitol, saccharin
	FD&C red #40, FD&C red #3	pharm. glaze	
	FD&C red #3, FD&C yellow #6, titanium dioxide		cane sugar, castor oil
	titanium dioxide, FD&C yellow #6	pharm. glaze	cane sugar
			cane sugar, art. cherry vanilla, sorbitol, saccharin
wheat starch			
		microcrystalline cellulose	cellulose
	FD&C yellow #10, FD&C yellow #6		
alcohol pres. or used in manufacture			

Product	Corn	Beef or Pork	Milk
Marion Labs Gaviscon liquid			
Marion Labs Gaviscon tablets	starch		
Marion Labs Gaviscon-2 tablets	starch		
Marion Labs Gly-Oxide liquid			
Marion Labs Nico-400 caps	starch		
Marion Labs Nitro-Bid caps	starch		
Marion Labs Nitro-Bid IV			
Marion Labs Os-Cal 500 tablets	starch, sugar		
Marion Labs Os-Cal Forte tabs	starch, sugar		
Marion Labs Os-Cal tablets	starch, sugar		
Marion Labs Ambenyl Expectorant	glucose		
Marion Labs Ambenyl-D			
Marion Labs Carafate tablets	starch		
Marion Labs Cardizem tablets 30 mg	starch		lactose
Marion Labs Ditropan syrup			
Marion Labs Ditropan tablets			lactose
Marion Labs Os-Cal-Gesic	starch, sugar		lactose
Marion Labs Pavabid caps	starch		
Marion Labs Pavabid HP capsules	starch		lactose

Wheat or Grains	Dyes	Gums and Resins	Miscellaneous
	FD&C yellow #10, FD&C blue #1		
			powdered cane sugar
			powdered cane sugar
alcohol pres. or used in manufacture			
alcohol pres. or used in manufacture			
alcohol pres. or used in manufacture			
alcohol pres. or used in manufacture	FD&C yellow #10, FD&C blue #1		
alcohol pres. or used in manufacture	FD&C yellow #10, FD&C blue #1		
alcohol pres. or used in manufacture	FD&C yellow #10, FD&C blue #1		
alcohol pres. or used in manufacture	FD&C red #33 FD&C red #40		sucrose from cane sugar
alcohol pres. or used in manufacture	FD&C red #40		sucrose from cane sugar
	FD&C blue #7, FD&C red #30		
	FD&C yellow #10, FD&C blue #1		
	FD&C green #3		sucrose from cane sugar
	FD&C blue #1		
	FD&C yellow #10, FD&B blue #1		Contains None of the Following: beet sugar, wheat, rice, yeast, soy, potato
alcohol pres. or used in manufacture			
alcohol pres. or used in manufacture			

237

Product	Corn	Beef or Pork	Milk
Marion Labs Throat Discs	starch		
Marion Labs Thyroid strong tabs (coated)	starch		
Marion Labs Thyroid strong tabs (plain)	starch		
Marion Labs Thyroid tablets	starch		
Marion Labs Triten 2.5 tablets	starch		lactose
Marion Labs Os-Cal Plus tabs	starch, sugar		
Marlyn Co. C-Speridin	zein, ascorbic acid		
Marlyn Co. Care-4	ascorbic acid	gelatin	
Marlyn Co. Hep Forte		gelatin, glycerine	
Marlyn Co. Marlyn Formula 50		gelatin, glycerine	
Marlyn Co. PMS	ascorbic acid	gelatin, glycerine	
Marlyn Co. Pro-Formance	ascorbic acid	gelatin	
Marlyn Co. Prolonged Release Vitamins			
Merell Dow Bentyl caps	starch	stearates	lactose
Merell Dow Bentyl syrup	glucose		
Merell Dow Bentyl tabs	starch, dextrose	stearates	lactose
Merell Dow Novafed A Liquid	gluconate, sucrose	glycerine	
Merell Dow Novafed Liquid	gluconate, invert sucrose	glycerine	
Merell Dow Novahistine cold tabs	starch		
Merell Dow Novahistine Cough Formula	gluconate	glycerine	
Merell Dow Novahistine elixir		glycerine	
Merell Dow Novahistine expectorant	gluconate	glycerine	
Merell Dow Novahistine Sinus tabs	starch	stearates	

Wheat or Grains	Dyes	Gums and Resins	Miscellaneous
			cane and powdered sugar
alcohol pres. or used in manufacture	FD&C yellow #6, FD&C blue #2, FD&C red #7		cane sugar
			cane sugar
			cane sugar
alcohol pres. or used in manufacture	FD&C yellow #5		sucrose from cane sugar
	FD&C red #19, FD&C red #33		
			citrus
	unspecified but present		vanillin, soy protein isolate, polysorbate 80
safflower oil			
	FD&C blue #1		
	FD&C yellow #6, FD&C red #40, FD&C blue #1, FD&C red #33		unspecified artificial flavors
	FD&B blue #1		
alcohol	FD&C yellow #10, FD&C blue #1		unspecified artificial flavors, sorbitol
alcohol	FD&C yellow #10, FD&C yellow #6, FD&C blue #1		unspecified artificial flavors, sorbitol
alcohol	FD&C red #40, FD&C blue #1		unspecified artificial flavors, sorbitol
alcohol	FD&C yellow #10, FD&C blue #1		unspecified artificial flavors, sorbitol
	FD&C red #40, FD&C yellow #10, FD&C blue #1		unspecified artificial flavors, sorbitol

Product	Corn	Beef or Pork	Milk
Merell Dow Tussend expectorant	gluconate, invert sucrose	glycerine	
Merell Dow Tussend liquid	invert sucrose	glycerine	
Merell Dow Tussend tabs	starch	stearates	
Miles Lab Flintstones & Bugs Bunny chewable tabs (also w/iron)	starch, ascorbic acid	gelatin, stearates, stearic acid	
Miles Lab One-A-Day Essential	ascorbic acid	gelatin, stearates	
Miles Lab One-A-Day Plus Iron	ascorbic acid	gelatin, stearates	
Miles Lab One-A-Day Plus minerals	starch, ascorbic acid	gelatin, stearates	
Miles Lab One-A-Day Stressgard and Plus Extra C	starch, ascorbic acid	gelatin, stearates	lactose
Norcliff Thayer "Keep Awake" tabs		stearic acid	lactose
Norcliff Thayer Amitone antacid	starch		
Norcliff Thayer Liquiprin Acetaminophen solution	syrup		
Norcliff Thayer Nature's Remedy laxative		stearates	lactose
Norcliff Thayer Tums—Lemon	starch		
Norcliff Thayer Tums—Cherry	starch		
Norcliff Thayer Tums—Extra Strength	starch		
Norcliff Thayer Tums—Orange	starch		
Norcliff Thayer Tums—Peppermint	starch		
Norcliff Thayer Tums—Wintergreen	starch		
Pennwalt Allerest caps	starch	stearates	lactose
Pennwalt Allerest chewable tabs		stearates	
Pennwalt Allerest tabs	starch	stearates	
Pennwalt Sinarest	starch	stearates	
Pfizer Laboratories Vistaril capsules	starch	stearates, gelatin	
Pfizer Laboratories Vistrax tabs	starch	stearates	lactose

Wheat or Grains	Dyes	Gums and Resins	Miscellaneous
alcohol	FD&C yellow #6		unspecified artificial flavors, sorbitol
alcohol	FD&C red #40		unspecified artificial flavors, sorbitol
	FD&C red #3, FD&C yellow #6		carnauba wax
	FD&C red #3 lake, FD&C yellow #6 lake, FD&C blue #2 lake		imit. grape, imit. raspberry, imit. strawberry, imit. cherry, imit. and natural orange and tangerine, imit.
	FD&C red #40 lake, FD&C yellow #6 lake, FD&C blue #2 lake		imit. vanilla, marshmallow
	FD&C yellow #5 lake, FD&C yellow #6 lake		imit. vanilla, marshmallow
	FD&C red #40 lake, FD&C yellow #6 lake, FD&C blue #2 lake		imit. vanilla, marshmallow flavors, yeast
	FD&C yellow #6 lake		imit. vanilla, marshmallow
			natural lemon
			nat. peppermint, talc
	FD&C red #3		art. raspberry
	FD&C yellow lake blend		nat. lemon, talc
	FD&C red #3		art. cherry, talc
	FD&C green lake blend		art. wintergreen, talc
	FD&C yellow #6		nat. orange, talc
			nat. peppermint, talc
	FD&C green lake blend		art. wintergreen, talc
starch	unspecified		unspecified flavorings, mannitol, sorbitol
	unspecified		talc
starch	unspecified		
	unspecified		sorbitol
	unspecified		sucrose (unspecified source)

Product	Corn	Beef or Pork	Milk
Pfizer Laboratories Diabinase tabs	starch	stearates	
Pfizer Laboratories Feldene caps	starch	gelatin, stearates	lactose
Pfizer Laboratories Minipress caps	starch	gelatin, stearates	
Pfizer Laboratories Minizide caps		stearates	
Pfizer Laboratories Moderil tabs	starch	stearates	lactose
Pfizer Laboratories Procardia			
Pfizer Laboratories Renese tabs	starch	stearates	lactose
Pfizer Laboratories Renese-R tabs	starch	stearates	lactose
Pfizer Laboratories Vibramycin caps	starch	gelatin	
Pfizer Laboratories Vibramycin susp	syrup		
Pfizer Laboratories Vibramycin syrup	syrup	gelatin	
Pfizer Laboratories Vibratabs		stearates	
Pfizer Laboratories Vistaril caps	starch	gelatin, stearates	
Pfizer Vistaril Oral susp	syrup		
Pharmacraft Div. Allerest tabs	starch	stearates	
Pharmacraft Div. Allerest caps	starch (?)	stearates	lactose
Pharmacraft Div. Allerest chewable tabs		stearates	
Pharmacraft Div. Sinarest tablets	starch (?)	stearates	
Reld-Provident Dentavite drops	ascorbic acid		
Reld-Provident Labs Quinik tabs			dicalcium phosphate
Reld-Provident Labs Bacarate tabs	starch		lactose
Reld-Provident Labs Histalet DM syrup			
Reld-Provident Labs Histalet Forte tabs	syrup, dextrose	stearic acid	lactose
Reld-Provident P.V. Tussin tabs	starch	stearic acid	lactose
Reld-Provident P.V. Tussin			
Reld-Provident RP-Mycin tabs	starch, dextrose	stearic acid	

Wheat or Grains	Dyes	Gums and Resins	Miscellaneous
	unspecified		
	unspecified		
	unspecified		sucrose (unspecified source)
	unspecified		sucrose (unspecified source)
	unspecified		
	unspecified		
	unspecified		
	unspecified		
			sucrose (unspecified source)
		unspecified	
	unspecified		
	unspecified		sucrose (unspecified source)
	unspecified		talc
starch (?)	unspecified		
	unspecified		unspecified flavors, mannitol, sorbitol
	unspecified		
			CF-58 Gentry art. fruit flavor, sorbitol
			magnesium stearate, cabosil
	FD&C red #3		magnesium stearate, cabosil
	FD&C yellow #6		imit. caramel #6, imit. raspberry, imit. cherry/rasp., imit. banana, imit. apricot
	FD&C blue #1, FD&C red #3		magnesium stearate, Corb-o-sil m5
	FD&C yellow #6	gelatin	talc, potato starch
alcohol	FD&C yellow #6		vanillin, sodium saccharin, imit. banana, sorbitol, citric acid
			talc, potato starch, magnesium stearate

Product	Corn	Beef or Pork	Milk
Reld-Provident tabs Dentavite tabs	ascorbic acid		
Reld-Provident Tusstrol	syrup		
Reld-Provident Unipres tabs	starch		lactose
Rondec T tabs	dextrose		
Ross Pediamycin products Ross Pediazole Ross Pramet FA	dextrose, glucose		
Ross Pramilet FA			
Ross Rondec S syrup	dextrose		
Ross Rondec T tabs	dextrose		
Ross Rondec TR	dextrose		lactose
Ross Rondec-DM drops & syrup	dextrose		
Ross ViDaylin (all)	dextrose, glucose		
Rowell C-Ron	ascorbic acid	magnesium stearate	
Rowell C-Ron FA	ascorbic acid	magnesium stearate	
Rowell C-Ron Forte	ascorbic acid	magnesium stearate	
Rowell C-Ron Freckles	ascorbic acid	magnesium stearate	
Rowell Cin-Quin caps	starch	gelatin (capsule), magnesium stearate	
Rowell Cin-Quin tabs		magnesium stearate	
Rowell Colrex Hydrocil Instant			
Rowell Colrex caps	modified starch	gelatin (cap), magnesium stearate	

Wheat or Grains	Dyes	Gums and Resins	Miscellaneous
			florasynth imit. cherry, talc, magnesium stearate, cabosil
	FD&C yellow #6		vanillin, nat. & art. cherry, florasynth, imit. cherry #3, citric acid
	FD&C yellow #6, FD&C yellow #10		
			synthetic alcohol used in preparation
(cane) sugar			
(cane) sucrose			
			synthetic alcohol used in preparation
			synthetic alcohol used in preparation
(cane) sucrose			
			synthetic alcohol used in preparation
			synthetic alcohol used in preparation
(cane) sucrose			synthetic alcohol used in preparation
			synthetic alcohol used in preparation, citrus
	FD&C yellow #6, FD&C blue #2, FD&C red #3		carnauba wax
	FD&C yellow #6, FD&C blue #2, FD&C red #3		carnauba wax, modified potato starch
	FD&C yellow #6, FD&C blue #2, FD&C red #3		carnauba wax, modified potato starch
	FD&C yellow #6 lake		mannitol, nat. & art. vanilla, art. orange
		acacia	modified potato starch
	FD&C red #3, FD&C yellow #6		

Product	Corn	Beef or Pork	Milk
Rowell Colrex compound caps	modified starch	gelatin (cap), magnesium stearate	
Rowell Colrex compound elixer		glycerine	
Rowell Colrex decongestant	starch	magnesium stearate	
Rowell Colrex Expectorant		glycerine	
Rowell Colrex Hydrocil Plain	dextrose		
Rowell Colrex Lithotabs		calcium stearate	
Rowell Colrex Lithowats		gelatin (capsule)	
Rowell Colrex Multivitamins	ascorbic acid	gelatin, glycerine	
Rowell Colrex syrup		glycerine	
Rowell Colrex Troches	syrup		
Rowell Norlac	ascorbic acid	magnesium stearate	
Rowell Norlac RX	ascorbic acid	magnesium stearate	
Rowell Orasone 1 (1 mg)		magnesium stearate	lactose
Rowell Orasone 10 (10 mg)		magnesium stearate	lactose
Rowell Orasone 20 (20 mg)		magnesium stearate	lactose
Rowell Orasone 5 (5 mg)		magnesium stearate	lactose
Rowell Orasone 50 (50 mg)		magnesium stearate	lactose
Rowell Vio-Bec	ascorbic acid	gelatin (cap), magnesium stearate	
Rowell Vio-Bec Forte	ascorbic acid	magnesium stearate	
Tyson Amino LAC			
Tyson Amino-Dox		stearates	
Tyson Amino-Vi-Min		stearates	
Tyson AminoB-Plex		stearates	
Tyson Aminoform caps		gelatin (cap)	
Tyson Aminoform powder			

Wheat or Grains	Dyes	Gums and Resins	Miscellaneous
	FD&C yellow #6, FD&C yellow #10		
alcohol	FD&C red #40, FD&C yellow #10, FD&C yellow #6		lemon, vanilla
alcohol	FD&C yellow #6		vanillin, carnauba wax
alcohol	FD&C yellow #10, FD&C yellow #6, FD&C blue #1		Gualferesin, sorbitol
			modified potato starch
	FD&C red #40		talc
	caramel		soybean oil, ethyl vanillin, yellow wax, sorbitol
alcohol	FD&C red #40, FD&C blue #1		wild cherry, sorbitol
	FD&C red #40		black currant
	FD&C red #3		modified potato starch, carnauba wax
	FD&C yellow #6		modified potato starch, carnauba wax
	FD&C red #3		modified potato starch
	FD&C blue #1		modified potato starch
	FD&C yellow #10		modified potato starch
			modified potato starch
			modified potato starch, carnauba wax
	FD&C yellow #6, FD&C blue #1, FD&C red #3		vanillin
	FD&C yellow #6, FD&C blue #2, FD&C red #3		carnauba wax
		guar gum	alfalfa, watercress, parsley, rose hips, bone meal, yeast, kelp, lecithin
food glaze, rice bran, alfalfa			yeast, rose hips, yeast

Product	Corn	Beef or Pork	Milk
Tyson AminoK		stearates	
Tyson Aminoplex caps		gelatin (cap)	
Tyson Aminoplex powder			
Tyson AminoZN		stearates	
Tyson Bromellen Forte		stearates	
Tyson Colloidal Trace Minerals		stearates	
Willen Drug Co. NeutraPhos-K Powder and caps			
Willen Drug Co. Polycitra-K syrup			
Willen Drug Co. Bicitra-Sugar Free			
Willen Drug Co. NeutraPhos Powder and caps			
Willen Drug Co. Polycitra syrup			
Willen Drug Co. Polycitra-LC-Sugar Free			
Winthrop-Breon Aralen tabs	starch, sucrose, glucose	gelatin, stearates	
Winthrop-Breon Bronkaid tabs	starch	stearates	
Winthrop-Breon Caroid tabs	sucrose	gelatin, stearates, stearic acid	lactose
Winthrop-Breon Demerol syrup	glucose		
Winthrop-Breon Demerol tabs	starch	stearic acid	
Winthrop-Breon Drisdol tabs		gelatin	
Winthrop-Breon Talwin compound tabs	starch	stearates	

Wheat or Grains	Dyes	Gums and Resins	Miscellaneous
	unspecified		unspecified flavorings, talc
	unspecified		unspecified flavorings
	unspecified	unspecified	unspecified flavorings
	unspecified		unspecified flavorings, talc
	unspecified		unspecified flavorings
	unspecified	unspecified	unspecified flavorings
	FD&C red #3	kaolin, acacia, beeswax, carnauba wax	talc
cellulose (avical)			
cellulose (avical)		acacia, beeswax, carnauba wax	silicon dioxide
			Benzoic acid, sod. saccharin, banana flavoring
			talc
	FD&C yellow #5, FD&C blue #1		soybean oil
cellulose (avical)			sodium lauryl sulfate

RESOURCES

MILK, CHEESES, AND SUBSTITUTES

(These are listed separately from the formulas as they do not contain additional vitamins and minerals.)

Goat Milk

Goat milk is available in three forms: fresh (usually in containers at health-food stores), evaporated and powdered.

JACKSON-MITCHELL PHARMACEUTICALS, INC.
800 Garden Street
Santa Barbara, CA 93108

Meyenberg Evaporated and Powdered Milk
Goat milk, plus the occasional stabilizers carageenan and disodium phosphate. (According to the company, these are "seldom used and then only in minute quantities. Both are present in all evaporated milks. . .".)

Goat's Milk Cheeses

The following cheeses are pure goat cheeses and can be found at specialty food stores. In some cases, they must be ordered.

Capricette – mild, creamy
Capricorne – sharp and dry
Chevrotin – fairly mild
Geant du Poitou – sharp
Montrachet – tart
Sant Saviol – quite rich

COLONY FOODS
P.O. Box 1275
Hawthorne, CA 90250

(Check with the company for the complete list of ingredients for the following products.)

Salt-free goat cheese
Goat cheddar

Powdered Soy Milk

There are many brands of flavored powdered soy milk on the market. In this list I am including only those which are made from 100% soy and contain no cow's milk. (Many of the "soy" milks contain cow's milk.) They should not be used as substitutes for infant's formula as they do not necessarily contain all of the nutrients which infants require for normal development.

ENER-G FOODS, INC.
P.O. Box 24723
Seattle, WA 98124

Jolly Joan Pure SoyQuick
Soy powder (Recipes for making whipped toppings and soy milk are on the back of the package, as are recipes for sour SoyQuik.) Contains no preservatives, sugar or artificial flavoring.

FEARN SOYA FOODS
Division of Richard Food Corporation
Melrose Park, IL 60160

Natural Soya Powder
Soybeans (Recipes are available from the manufacturer or at health food stores.) Solvents and chemicals are not used in the manufacture of the soy powder. *Note:* On the manufacturer's product fact sheet, there is a notice not to use the powder in the diet of infants under 1 year of age unless recommended by a physician.

Low-Fat Soya Powder
Soybeans (above) with the soybean oil removed by pressing.

EL MOLINO MILLS
345 Baldwin Park Blvd.
City of Industry, CA 91796

Soya Powder (for milk)
soybeans

Fresh Soy Milk

Soy milk has been manufactured for more than 2000 years in China. More recently discovered as a source of protein in this country, it can be produced in many forms.

The Chinese method of making soy milk produces a liquid with a nutty or beany flavor. It is served in bowls and drunk, with the addition of sugar or other flavoring.

Members of the Food Science and Technology Department of Cornell University, Professors Hand, Wilkins, Mattick, Lo, and Steinkraus, developed a method of manufacturing soy milk which eliminated many of the components of the milk which produce the "beany" taste. It was these components which had previously made soy milk unacceptable to many people. They have graciously made the method available to the public. The method is as follows:

1. Wash and sort the beans to remove dirt and damaged soybeans.

2. Soak 1/2 cup of soybeans 6 hours or overnight in 3 times their weight water, at room temperature.

3. Drain and rinse the soybeans with progressively hotter water.

4. Divide the beans into equal portions.

5. Preheat blender jar with first hot water, then boiling water. If the jar is glass, bring the temperature up in several steps to avoid cracking.

6. Place 1 portion of the beans in the blender jar and add 2 cups of boiling water. Cover the blender top with a thick towel or hot-pot holder, and be sure to use a protective mit on the hand holding down the top. (Do this to avoid boiling water spillage.) Blend for 3 minutes. In order to eliminate the beany flavor, the beans and water must be kept above 180°F throughout the grinding process.

7. This slurry is then forced through a jelly bag or fine mesh to produce the milk.

8. Add 2 more cups water to the beans, reprocess them in the blender, and force the mixture through the jelly bag again.

According to the developers of this technique, the resulting milk has approximately the same protein content as cow's milk, depending on the soybeans used, with a lower calcium content. Calcium content can be increased by fortification.

The fat content can be increased by the addition of oil, and at this stage, flavorings may be added.

To each quart of milk, you may add one of the following:

oil	2-4 teaspoons
sugar	1 tablespoon
vanilla	1 teaspoon
coconut milk	1 1/2 fluid ounces
carob powder	2 teaspoons

Health Valley
Flavored soy milk, called Soymoo, containing honey, vegetable fat, natural flavoring and sea salt. It contains no preservatives and is sold frozen)

See the Children's Special section for soy based formulas.

Soy Cheese or Tofu

Tofu is fermented soy milk, producing a bland moist cheese which is used in Oriental cooking. It easily absorbs flavors, and can be prepared in many ways. (See Recipe section.) It is available at most Oriental food stores, health food stores, and can often be found in the produce section of supermarkets. Commercially-made tofu sometimes contains lactic, tartaric or citric acid.

To make tofu from soybeans you need:

1 cup dry soybeans
4 cups water
1 1/2 teaspoons nigari or juice of 1 lemon

Follow the method for making soy milk, using the amount of water stated above. Place 2 layers of cheese cloth in a colander which is then placed over a bowl. Mix the nigari or lemon juice in a cup of hot water. Bring the soymilk to a boil, reduce the heat and simmer, stirring, for 5 minutes. Stir in 1/2 the nigari or lemon juice solution and allow to sit for several minutes. Gently sprinkle the rest of the solution over the top of the milk and allow to sit, covered, until the curds form. When milk is entirely separated, moisten the cheesecloth and gently ladle milk into it. Fold the edges of the cloth up, place a pound weight on top and allow the milk to drip through. When the cloth stops dripping, turn the tofu out gently into the whey solution and refrigerate.

MEATS

In most areas of the country, there are meat and poultry producers who raise their stock without use of hormones or drugs, and who package their products without added ingredients. They are usually small producers and the consumer can best discover their names by asking at local health food stores. Lately, however, many larger producers have begun publicizing the fact that they do not use hormones or drugs. This information is easily obtained by writing to the producer, as the address usually appears on the package, or can be provided by the meat department of your local store.

Processed Meats

There are many imitation and/or processed meats now available at the market. It is important to note however, that many of them contain ingredients which you may be trying to avoid.

HEALTH VALLEY NATURAL FOODS
Los Angeles, CA 90021

Uncured Cooked Sausage made with Chicken or Turkey
Weiner flavoring added. Chicken (or turkey), water, salt, natural spices, paprika, fresh onions, lemon juice, fresh garlic

Jumbo Cooked Beef Sausage
Beef, water, salt, natural spices, fresh onions, fresh garlic, lemon juice

Chub Cooked Beef Sausage
Beef, water, salt, natural spices, fresh onions, fresh garlic, lemon juice

Cooked Beef Dinner Sausage
Beef, water, salt, natural spices, fresh onions, fresh garlic, lemon juice

Pork Link Sausage (skinless)
Pork, salt, natural spices (not specified), honey

Liver Sausage
Pork liver, pork, beef, nonfat dry milk, onions, water, salt, flavorings.

SHELTON'S POULTRY INC.
Pomona, CA 91767

Chick-a-dee's cooked uncured Chicken Franks
No nitrates or nitrites. Chicken, sea salt, unspecified spices

Meat Substitutes

WORTHINGTON FOODS DIVISION OF MILES
LABORATORIES
Worthington, OH 43085

Sliced Soyameat (artificial beef flavor)
Water, textured spun soy protein (fibrotein), corn oil, wheat flour, egg white solids, partially hydrogenated cottonseed and coconut oils, yeast extract, modified corn starch, natural flavorings from nonfat sources, caramel color, soy sauce, corn syrup solids, salt, onion powder, monosodium glutamate, niacin, iron (as ferrous sulfate), disodium inosinate/disodium guaylate, artificial colors, thiamine, Vitamin B, riboflavin, Vitamin B_{12}. Kosher, pareve

Sliced Soyameat (artificial chicken flavor)
Water, textured spun soy protein (fibroprotein), corn oil, egg white solids, hydrolyzed vegetable protein, modified corn starch, soy protein salt, natural flavorings from nonfat sources, monosodium glutamate, onion powder, spices, carageenan, niacin, iron (as ferrous sulfate), thiamine, Vitamin B, artificial color, riboflavin and Vitamin B_{12}. Kosher, pareve

Numete, a vegetable protein product
Water peanuts, corn and soy flour, salt, monosodium glutamate, niacin, thiamine, iron (as ferrous sulfate), Vitamin B, riboflavin, Vitamin B_{12}. Kosher, pareve

Chili
Water, red beans, wheat protein, tomato paste, corn oil, soy sauce, modified corn starch, salt, dehydrated onions, sugar, monosodium glutamate, caramel color yeast extract, hydrolyzed vegetable protein, garlic powder, mushrooms, dextrose, artificial flavorings from nonfat sources, niacin, iron (as ferrous sulfate), thiamine, Vitamin B, riboflavin, Vitamin B_{12}. Kosher, pareve

FriChik
Soyameat (vegetable product – artificial fried chicken flavor) water, spun soy protein (fibroprotein), soybean and corn oil, egg white solids, hydrolyzed vegetable protein, modified corn starch, soy protein, salt, monosodium glutamate, natural flavorings from nonmeat sources, onion powder, carrageenen, niacinamide, iron (as ferrous sulfate), Vitamin B, (pyridoxine hydrochloride), artificial color, Vitamin B (riboflavin) and Vitamin B_{12} (Cyanocobalamin). Kosher, pareve

Protos (a vegetable protein product)
Wheat protein, water, peanuts, wheat flour, corn oil, yeast extract, soy sauce, salt, hydrolyzed vegetable protein, niacin, iron, thiamine, Vitamin B, riboflavin, Vitamin B_{12}. Kosher, pareve

Granburger (dehydrated)
Soy protein concentrate, isolated soy protein, textured spun soy protein (Fibroprotein), onion powder, hydrolyzed vegetable protein, sugar, salt, artificial color, niacinamide, iron (as ferrous sulfate), artificial flavor from nonmeat sources, D-Calcium pantothenate, Vitamin B_6 (pyridoxine hydrochloride), Vitamin B_2 (riboflavin), Vitamin B_1 (thiamine mononitrite), and Vitamin B_{12} (cyanocobalamin)

Note: The caramel coloring in Worthington products is made from burnt sugar.

LOMA LINDA FOODS
Riverside, CA 92505

Proteena

Wheat gluten, raw peanut butter, water, tomato puree, soy flour, salt, yeast extract, hydrolyzed vegetable protein, L-Lysine, caramel coloring, vitamins, onion powder, spices, iron sulfate.

Vege-Burger

Wheat gluten, water, soy flour, salt, natural flavors of vegetable origin, caramel color, dextrose, onion powder, L-Lysine, niacinamide, thiamine mononitrate, D-calcium pantothenate, pyridoxine hydrochloride, riboflavin, cyancocobalamin. Kosher, pareve

Linketts

Wheat gluten, soy oil, water, dried yeast, salt, soy protein concentrate, natural vegetable and artificial flavors, soy flour, vegetable mono- and di-glycerides, soy lecithin, L-Lysine, onion powder, caramel color, artificial color, garlic powder, niacinamide, D-calcium pantothenate, thiamine, mono-nitrate, pyridoxine hydrochloride, riboflavin, cyanocobalamin. Kosher, pareve

Chili

Water, pinto beans, tomato puree, textured soy granules, soy oil, salt, paprika, chili powder, natural flavor, wheat flavor, onion powder, sugar, garlic powder, lecithin. Kosher, pareve

Nuteena

Raw peanut butter, soy flour, corn flour, rice flour, dried yeast, salt, yeast extract, onion powder, L-Lysine, hydrolyzed vegetable protein, di-Methionine, natural flavoring.

Vita-Burger (meatless textured soy granules)

Soy flour, salt, natural flavor of vegetable origin, caramel color, artificial flavor, spices, niacinamide, ferris sulfate, D-calcium

FEARN SOYA FOODS
Division of Richards Food Corporation
Melrose Park, IL 60160

Soya Granules
Soybeans

Sesame Burger Mix
Sesame meal, soy flour, raw wheat germ, dry roasted soybeans, nutritional yeast, dried tamari, soy sauce, dried miso, water washed wheat gluten, dulse, garlic powder, onion, parsley, celery seeds, herbs. No texturized vegetable protein, no preservatives.

Beef and Veal

HEALTH VALLEY NATURAL FOODS
Los Angeles, CA 90021

Health Maid Meats
Beef fed on natural grass and clover. Supplementary feeding includes safflower, soybeans, wheat germ, oil, vitamins and other natural diet. Also sorgum, kelp, cider, vinegar, flax and raisin meal. They are not fed DES.

Like most meats in health food stores, Health Valley sliced beef liver (8 oz. package) is sold frozen.

TEEL MOUNTAIN FARM
Box 550
Standardsville, VA 22973

Veal and Baby Beef
The veal is milk-fed calf from non-weaned calves. (No growth stimulants or milk replacers.) The baby beef are also non-weaned calves which weigh around 240 lbs, and have red meat. The mothers are grazed in the field and are not fed DES, pesticides or antibiotics. The meat is aged, frozen, and guaranteed for safe arrival.

FLOURS AND FLOUR MIXES

FEARN SOYA FOODS
4520 James Place
Melrose Park, IL 60160

Rice Flour
Finely ground rice from which the bran and hull have been removed. Recipes are on the package.

Soy-O Rice Baking Mix
Rice flour, soya powder, dextrose, calcium phosphate, sodium bicarbonate, salt, vegetable gum

Low Fat Soya Powder
Soybeans

ENER-G FOODS, INC.
P.O. Box 24723
Seattle, WA 98124

Recipes are on the packages.

Pure Rice Flour
Rice Flour. No preservatives or artificial flavorings.

Rice Bran
Defatted rice bran. No preservatives or artificial flavorings.

Rice Polish
Rice polish is the flour taken off the brown rice in order to make white rice. No preservatives or artificial flavorings.

Rice Mix
Rice flour, rice starch, rice polish, cereal-free baking powder, salt. No preservatives or artificial flavorings.

Rice 'n Rye Bread Mix
Rice flour, rye flour, sea salt, baking powder.

Barley Mix
Barley flour, leavening and sea salt.

Oat Mix
Oat flour, cereal-free baking powder, salt. No preservatives or artificial flavorings.

Potato Mix
Potato flour, cereal-free baking powder, salt. No preservatives or flavoring added.

CELLU
Chicago Dietetic Supply, Inc.
P.O. Box 40
LaGrange, IL 60525

Recipe folders are included in each package of flour.

Cellu Potato Starch
Potato starch

Cellu Wheat Starch
Wheat starch

Cellu Tapioca Starch
Tapioca starch

EL MOLINO MILLS
345 Baldwin Park Blvd.
City of Industry, CA 91746

Buckwheat, corn and soya flour; corn meal

B. MANISCHEWITZ COMPANY
Jersey City, NJ 07302

Potato Starch

ARGO
Best Foods
Inglewood Cliffs, NJ 07632

Argo Corn Starch

KODA FARMS, INC.
South Dos Palos, CA 93665

Mochiko Sweet Rice Flour, Blue Star Brand

CEREAL-FREE BAKING POWDER

CELLU
Chicago Dietetic Supply, Inc.
P.O. Box 40
La Grange, IL 60525

Cellu Cereal-Free Baking Powder
Potato starch, phosphate of calcium, sodium bicarbonate

BREADS

FOOD FOR LIFE BAKING COMPANY, INC.
3580 N. Pasadena Avenue
Los Angeles, CA 90031

100% Wheat-Free, Gluten-Free, Rice Bread
Rice flour, water, honey, soya oil, natural gum, fresh yeast, salt

100% Wheat-Free White Rye Bread
White rye flour, water, honey, molasses, fresh yeast, soya oil, lecithin, malt.

GIUSTO'S SPECIALTY FOODS
241 East Harris Avenue
South San Francisco, California 94080

Bray's Formula Breads:

Soya Potato Bread
Soya flour, potato starch, water, soya oil, leavening*, sugar, salt

Rice Bread
Rice flour, potato starch, soya flour, water, soya oil, sugar, leavening*, salt

Lima Bean Bread
Soya flour, potato starch, lima bean flour, water, sugar, leavening*, salt

Leavening: Bray's baking powder (sodium pyrophosphate, soda bicarbonate, potato starch)

ENER-G FOODS, INC.
P.O. Box 84487
6901 Fox Avenue South
Seattle, WA 98124-5787

White Rice Yeast-Free Bread
White rice flour, water, safflower oil, Methylcellulose, baking powder(glucono-delta-lactone, sodium bicarbonate), gelatin, calcium propionate.

COOKIES AND CAKES

EL MOLINO MILLS
Division of ACG Company
City of Industry, CA 91746

Carob Wheat-Free Old Fashioned Cookies
Barley flour, dark brown sugar, vegetable shortening, carob powder, whole eggs, lecithin, pure vanilla, baking soda, salt, baking powder

Cara Coa'n Rice Snack
Brown rice, partially hardened vegetable oil, fructose, carob powder, nonfat dry milk powder, soy oil, whole milk powder, sesame seed, lecithin, natural flavors.

HEALTHWAY INDUSTRIES
South San Francisco, CA 94080

Rice Applesauce Honey-Sweetened Cookies
Rice flour, partially hydrogenated soybean oil, honey unsweetened applesauce, spices, baking powder.

CHICO SAN INC.
1144 West First Street
Chico, CA 95926

San-Wich
Brown rice, sesame seeds, Chico San Yinnies syrup (brown rice and barley sweetener), oat flour, agar-agar, sesame oil, lecithin

CELLU
Chicago Dietetic Supply, Inc.
P.O. Box 40
LaGrange, IL 60525

Cellu Rye Bread
Yeast bread. Rye flour, water cottonseed shortening, cane sugar, yeast, salt

Master All-Rye Wafers
Whole rye flour and water

Cellu Rice Wafers
Whole grain rice and water

Feather River Rice Cakes
Puffed whole grain rice and sesame seeds (available salted and unsalted).

Cellu Wheat-Free Cake
Mandioca flour (like tapioca), cane sugar, cottonseed shortening, eggs, salt, vanilla and almond flavoring.

CRACKERS

Rye-Crisp™ and AK-MOK™ rye crackers are available at most supermarkets and are egg, milk, and wheat free.

HOL GRAIN DIVISION, GOLDEN GRAIN
Seattle, WA 98103

Hol-Grain Natural Rice Wafer-ets (salted or unsalted)
Contain natural brown rice, water and salt.

GOLDEN HARVEST
Natural Sales Company
Pittsburgh, PA 15203

Whole Grain Rice Waferetts
Natural brown rice, water, salt

KITANIHON CONFECTIONERY COMPANY, LTD.

Plain Rice Crunch Crackers
Rice, sea salt, soybean, oil

KA-ME (INTERSALES INC., U.S.A. SALES
REPRESENTATIVE)
West Nyack, NY 10994

Rice Crackers
Rice, sea salt, vegetable oil

CHICO SAN INC.
1144 West First Street
Chico, CA 95926

Rice Cakes, several varieties:

1. Rice cakes, unsalted – whole brown rice, sesame seeds.
2. Whole brown rice, sesame seeds and salt
3. Whole brown rice, millet, sesame seeds and salt
4. Whole brown rice, buckwheat, sesame seeds and salt

GARDEN ORGANICS
99 Pond Road
Asheville, NC 28806

Rice Cakes, several varieties:
1. Rice (brown)
2. Rice and salt
3. Rice and sesame
4. Rice, sesame and salt

STARCH PRODUCTS

The following noodle products can be found in Chinese, Korean, and/or Japanese food stores:

Rice Sticks
These are of varying widths, from thin spaghetti to wider noodles.

Bean Starch Sticks
These are usually of the thin variety, and the bean starch comes from different beans, labelled on the packages.

Bean Starch or Rice Sheets
Large round sheets which can be soaked and cut to any desired width or shape

Soba
Buckwheat noodles

Aproten Low Protein Diet Products
Noodles and macaroni made without wheat flour or eggs

CELLU
Chicago Dietetic Supply, Inc.
P.O. Box 40
La Grange, IL 60525

Rigatini, Tagliatelle, Anellini, Semolina, Noodle products
Cornstarch, tapioca starch, microcrystalline cellulose, and artificial color.

GENTILI AGLUTELLA (distributed by Ener-G Foods, Inc.)
6901 Fox Avenue South
P.O. Box 24723
Seattle, WA 98124

Spaghetti, Macaroni, Spaghetti Rings and Tagliatelle
Cornstarch, rice and potato starch, monoglycerides, carotene

FOOD FOR LIFE BAKING COMPANY, INC.
3580 Pasadena Avenue
Los Angeles, CA 90031

Wheat-Free Rice Elbow Macaroni
Brown rice flour, carbohydrate gum

CANNED FRUITS

CELLU
Chicago Dietetic Supply, Inc.
P.O. Box 40
La Grange, IL 60525

Fruits packed under the featherweight labels are processed without the addition of sweeteners of any type. Juice pack is red-labeled, and water pack is blue labeled. They contain no corn, beet or cane sugar.

EGG SUBSTITUTES

ENER-G FOODS, INC.
P.O. Box 24723
Seattle, WA 98124

Ener-G™ Egg Replacer
Arrowroot flour, potato starch, tapioca flour, modified vegetable gums, cereal-free leavening

SWEETENERS

ALLIED OLD ENGLISH, INC.
100 Markley Street
Port Reading, NJ 07064

Blackstrap molasses (See Food Charts for nutrients)
Barbados molasses, unsulphured

LANDSTROM COMPANY
Healthway brand
P.O. Box 2886
South San Francisco, CA 94080

Distributes many kinds of honeys, unblended, uncooked and unfiltered which are all labeled organic, such as: lemon honey, alfalfa honey, apple honey, carrot honey, sage honey, clover honey, etc.

AMERICAN MAPLE PRODUCTS
Newport, VT 05855

Maple sugar, in hard cakes and granulated
Maple sugar candy
Maple syrup (pure)
100% maple butter (fondant of syrup containing no butter)

They also sell maple blend candy and syrups so be sure to specify exactly what you want.

COOMBS BEAVER BROOK SUGARHOUSE
Box 503
Jct. Rts. 9 & 100
Wilmington, VT 05363

Note: Vermont maple syrup is graded under the Maple Syrup Grading Law which mandates it to be free of preservatives.

Maple syrup (pure) 3 grades
Pure maple candy
Old fashioned grained sugar
Granulated maple sugar
Maple cream
Maple blend candies

A book of recipes for the use of maple sweeteners is available from the University of Vermont, Extension Service, Burlington, Vermont (circular 137) for 25 cents.

NUT BUTTERS

HAIN PURE FOOD COMPANY
13660 South Figueroa Street
Los Angeles, CA 90061

Raw Blanched Almond Butter
Roasted Blanched Almond Butter
Raw Unblanched Almond Butter
Raw Cashew Butter
Roasted Cashew Butter
Peanut Sesame Butter
Raw Peanut Butter
Raw Sesame Butter
Sunflower Seed Butter
Creamy Peanut Butter
Crunchy Peanut Butter
Creamy Peanut Butter lightly salted
Crunchy Peanut Butter lighly salted

OILS

HAIN PURE FOOD COMPANY
13660 South Figueroa Street
Los Angeles, CA 90061

These oils have no other ingredients added.

Almond oil
Apricot oil
Avocado oil
Coconut oil
Cod liver oil
Corn oil
Cottonseed oil
Linseed oil
Olive oil
Peanut oil
Rice bran oil

Safflower oil
Sesame oil
Soy oil
Sunflower oil
Walnut oil
Wheat germ oil

Crude oils - Hain Pure Food Company
Corn oil
Peanut oil
Pumpkin Seed oil
Safflower oil
Sesame oil
Soy oil

FRUIT JUICES

COLONY FOODS
P.O. Box 1275
Hawthorne, CA 90250

These are frozen fresh, with no sugar or preservatives added.
Apple
Grape
Apricot-Pineapple
Boysenberry-Apple
Coconut-Pineapple
Peach-Apple
Banana-Apple
Strawberry-Apple
Raspberry
Papaya

HAIN PURE FOOD COMPANY, INC.
13660 South Figueroa Street
Los Angeles, CA 90061

These contain no additional ingredients.

Apple juice, filtered
Apple juice, unfiltered
Apricot juice
Blackberry juice
Black Cherry juice
Blueberry juice
Boysenberry juice
Fig juice w/lemon
Grape juice
Pomegranate juice
Prune juice w/lemon
Red Raspberry juice
Red Cherry juice

Hain also has a line of fruit concentrates: apple apricot, blackberry, black cherry, cranberry, plum, strawberry, and red raspberry.

NON-ANIMAL GELATIN

EMES KOSHER GELATIN
4138-42 West Roosevelt Road
Chicago, IL 60624

Depending on the flavor of the particular product, their gelatin contains: sugar, pareve gelatin, irish moss extract, locust bean gum, cotton gum, soya protein (fortified), citric acid, natural flavor, artificial flavor, color (all vegetable except lime). They also make unflavored gelatin.

HIME BRAND
Japan Food Corporation
San Francisco, CA 94080

Agar-Agar Square Fancy
Preparation directions are on the package.

271

CARMEL KOSHER FOOD PRODUCTS
Douglas Food Corporation
4840 South Kedzie Avenue
Chicago, IL 60632

Unflavored kosher gelatin
Various flavored gelatins (The strawberry contains: sugar, dextrose, kosher gelatin, citric acid, sodium citrate, salt, artificial flavor and artificial color.)
Low calorie gelatin dessert (The orange contains: kosher gelatin, citric acid, calcium, saccharin, ammoniated glycyrrhizin, artificial flavor, artificial color. The box bears a warning on saccharin.)

SOUPS AND GRAVIES

HEALTH VALLEY NATURAL FOODS
Los Angeles, CA 90021

Various soups packaged in enamel-lined cans.

CARMEL FOODS
Douglas Food Corporation
4840 South Kedzie Avenue
Chicago, IL 60632

Powdered soups – They are kosher and pareve, some with meat-like flavors. (This means that there is no pork, no milk, no meat.)
Powdered gravies – with the above considerations.

ADDITIONAL RECIPES
AND RESOURCES

The industry-sponsored pamphlets are free. Some of the others are available for a fee.

Allergy Diets
Ralston Purina Company
Nutrition Service
Checkerboard Square
St. Louis, MO 63164   recipes

Baking for People with Food Allergies
Supt. of Documents
U.S. Government Printing Office
Washington, D. C. 20402   recipes

Best Foods
Division of CPC International, Inc.
International Plaza
Englewood Cliffs, NJ 07632   recipes

California Apricot Advisory Board
1295 Boulevard Way
Suite H
Walnut Creek, CA 94595   recipes and nutrition info.

California Raisin Advisory Board
P.O. Box 5335
Fresno, CA 93755   recipes and nutrition info.

California Turkey Industry Federation
14th Street
Modesto, CA 95354   recipes and nutrition info.

Cara Coa
El Molino Mills
City of Industry, CA 91746   recipes

Diets Unlimited for Limited Diets
Allergy Information Association
3 Powburn Place
Weston 627 Ontario Canada   recipes and information

Easy Appealing Recipes (Milk-Free)
Mead Johnson Laboratories
Department 852
Evansville, IN 47721   recipes

Ener-G Foods Inc.
1526 Utah Avenue South
Box 24723
Seattle, WA 98124   recipes

Gerber
Department 54-3
445 State Street
Fremont, MI   product information

Good Eating for the Milk-Sensitive Person
Ross Laboratories
625 Cleveland Avenue
Columbus, OH 43216   recipes

125 Great Recipes for Allergy Diets
Good Housekeeping
969 Eighth Avenue
New York, NY 10019   recipes

Plantation
Allied Old English, Inc.
100 Markley Street
Port Reading, NJ 07064   recipes (molasses)

Presto Food Products, Inc.
929 East 14th Street
Los Angeles, CA 90021   recipes for Mocha Mix

Sunsweet Prune Kitchen
P.O. Box 26663
San Francisco, CA 94126   recipes and info.

Temeco West
Sun Giant
Box 9380
Bakersfield, CA 93309   recipes and product info.

Worthington Foods
Division of Miles Laboratory, Inc.
900 Proprietors Road
Worthington, OH 43085   recipes for meat substitutes

MAIL ORDER RESOURCES

Pavo's
57 South Ninth Street
Minneapolis, MN 55402

Provides an extensive catalog containing nationally known
health foods and apparatus, plus vitamins, dried foods, etc.

Better Foods Foundation, Inc.
300 North Washington Street
Greencastle, PA 17225

Catalog of health food items, vitamins, honey etc.

Jaffe Brothers
P.O. Box 636
Valley Center, CA 92082

Catalog of dried and fresh fruit, grains, nuts and honey.

The Garden Way Country Kitchen Catalog
1186 Williston Road
South Burlington, VT 05401

Catalog of kitchen, canning, and garden utensils. Many
hard-to-find items.

Lekvar-by-the-Barrel
1577 First Avenue
New York, NY 10028

Catalog of gourmet foods, nuts, beans, peas, rice, spices, herbs,
cooking utensils.

BIBLIOGRAPHY

Aas, Kjell, M.D. *The Allergic Child*. Springfield, IL, 1971.

Breneman, James C. *Basics of Food Allergy*. Springfield,IL: Thomas, 1978.

Catsimpoolas, Nicholas. *Immunological Aspects of Foods*. Westport, CT: Avi Publishing, 1977.

Coca, Arthur, M.D., et al. *Familial Nonreagenic Food Allergy*. Springfield, IL: Thomas, 1953.

Collins-Williams, Cecil. *Pediatric Allergy and Clinical Immunology (as applied to Atopic Disease): A Manual for Students and Practitioners of Medicine*. Toronto, 1973.

Criep, Leo H., M.D. *Allergy and Clinical Immunology*. New York: Grune and Stratton, 1976.

Delmont, J. ed. *Milk Intolerances and Rejection*. New York: Karger Press, 1982.

Eagle, Robert. *Eating and Allergy*. Garden City, NY: Random House, 1981.

Feingold, B.F., M.D. *Why your Child is Hyperactive*. New York: Random House, 1975.

Frazier, Claude A., M.D. *Parent's Guide to Allergy in Children*. New York: Grosset and Dunlap, 1978.

----------. *Coping with Food Allergy*. New York: New York Times/ Quadrangle Book, 1974.

Gerrard, J.W. *Food Allergy: New Perspectives*. Springfield, MA: Thomas, 1980. (includes index and bibliography)

Lessof, ed. *Clinical Reactions to Food*. New York: Wiley, 1983.

Patterson, Roy, M.D. *Allergic Diseases, Diagnosis and Management.* Philadelphia: Lippencott, 1972.

Rowe, Albert H., M.D. *Food Allergy, Its Manifestations, Diagnosis and Treatment.* Philadelphia, 1932.

Speer, Frederic, M.D. et al. *The Allergic Child.* New York, 1966.

-------------. *Food Allergy.* Boston: J. Wright/PSG, 1983.

Taube, E. Louis, M.D. *Food Allergy and the Allergic Patient.* Springfield, IL, 1973.

U.S. Department of Agriculture Handbook #8, Composition of Foods

Wunderlich, Ray C., M.D. *Allergy, Brains, and Children Coping.* St. Petersburg, FL: Johnny Reads, 1973

Winter, Ruth. *A Consumer's Dictionary of Food Additives.* New York: Crown, 1978.

RECIPE INDEX

Codes: C - Citrus, M - Meat or Animal Products (including Seafood), D - Dairy Products, W - Wheat, G - Grains other than Wheat, E - Eggs. Parentheses ( ) indicate that there are alternatives: for instance, wheat or another grain may be used, or perhaps there is a non-grain alternative, pareve gelatin may be used, egg substitutes may be used, or a number of alternatives may be available for dairy products. In recipes using packaged mixes, we did not attempt to evaluate all the ingredients in the mix since they do change. We advise that you carefully check all ingredient panels and contact the manufacturer if you are unsure about what is included..

The Cruise Answer Book: A Comprehensive Guide to the S.
of North America by Charlanne F. Herring. This book offers a
amount of information about ships, itineraries, shore excursions, an
is not included in other cruise guides, and that will help you decide wh
is best for you at any particular time. This book concentrates on cruise.
North America, the Caribbean, Bermuda, Hawaii...the areas where
Americans choose to cruise. **$9.95**

Adventure Traveling: Where the Packaged Tours Won't Take You by T.
"Tex" Hill. Whether you're looking for the keen edge of real danger or trips
that invoke the tingle without the threat, here's an international menu of
itineraries and guidelines for the vacationer who is looking for a "different"
kind of vacation. **$9.95**

Order Form

If you are unable to find our books in your local bookstore, you may order them
directly from us. Please enclose check or money order for amount of purchase
plus handling charge of $1.00 per book.

( ) Winning Tactics for Women Over Forty @$9.95 _____

( ) Aquacises @$9.95   _____

( ) There ARE Babies to Adopt @$9.95   _____

( ) Fifty and Fired! @$9.95   _____

( ) Your Astrological Guide to Fitness @$9.95   _____

( ) Bachelor in The Kitchen @$7.95   _____

( ) 60-Second Shiatzu @$7.95   _____

( ) Smart Travel @$9.95   _____

( ) The Cruise Answer Book @$9.95   _____

( ) Adventure Traveling @$9.95   _____

   Add $1.00 per book handling charge   _____

   Add 5% Sales Tax if MA resident   _____

   Total Amount enclosed   _____

Name _____

Address _____

City/State/Zip_____

Mail to: Mills & Sanderson, Publishers
         442 Marrett Road, Suite 5
         Lexington, MA 02173

Other Books from Mills & Sanderson

**Winning Tactics for Women Over Forty: How to Take Charge of
and Have Fun Doing It** by Anne DeSola Cardoza and Mavis B. Sutton
faceted guide for those women now in their forties and fifties who have
found themselves having to adapt their lifestyles to a world for which
not prepared. Explicit chapters cover such essentials as health, person
adapting to loss, financial planning, housing options, etc. The cor
techniques, resources and options available to these women are e
covered. **$9.95**

Aquacises: Restoring and Maintaining Mobility with Water Exe
Miriam Study Giles. Unlike most of the exercise books presently availa
cises is devoted to both the physical and psychological fitness of thos
who just want to feel better—and move around better in their normal
Written by a former dancer who has taught swimming and exercise
than half a century, this book is primarily focused on senior citize
but is also an invaluable resource for those suffering from physical
and those too self-conscious about their shapes to join in community ca
$9.95

There ARE Babies to Adopt: A Resource Guide for Prospective P
Christine A. Adamec. Author-researcher Adamec, an adoptive paren
provides a tremendous amount of valuable information and advice
helping you adopt the baby you want. Gleaned from both personal e
and in-depth interviews with over a hundred other adoptive pare
workers, and other adoption specialists, this practical guidebook dispe
ular myth that there are no healthy babies available for adoption
are willing to wait five to seven years. **$9.95**

Fifty and Fired! How to Prepare for It; What to Do When It H
Ed Brandt with Leonard Corwen. The authors lead the middle-age
manager through the trauma of age motivated job dismissal using ac
hitting case histories to show what can be done before and after
defend your career and dignity, and rebuild your livelihood. **$9.9**

Your Astrological Guide to Fitness by Eva Shaw. Find out what
logical sign has to say about your ideal exercises, sports, and menus.
also astrologically keyed gift ideas and comparison charts to help
your ideal mate or traveling companion. **$9.95**

Bachelor in The Kitchen: Beyond Bologna and Cheese by Gord
with Wendy Haskett. From Beer Jello to Duck with Cherries, San
Gordon Haskett shows you quick and easy recipes for yourself and/or
someone in your life; also, how to be the hit of any party or Pot L

60-Second Shiatzu: How to Energize, Erase Pain, and Conquer
One Minute by Eva Shaw. The author explains how acupressure re
self-administered amidst the frustrations of commuter rush hours, col
family fights, or office hassles. It's fun, it's easy, and it works! **$7**

**Smart Travel: Trade Secrets for Getting There in Style at Litt
Effort** by Martin Blinder. The author's thirty years of globe-span
have taught him many secrets for getting the best of everything
expense as feasible, and he wants to share those secrets with yo